EATING FOR ENDURANCE

Dr. Philip Maffetone

A sensible approach to diet and nutrition for the endurance athlete

The information contained in this book is from the author's experiences and is not intended to replace medical advice. It is not the intent of the author to diagnose or prescribe. Before beginning any program you should consult with your physician, and address any questions to your physician.

Case studies in this book are those of real people whose names have been changed to protect their confidentiality.

Editor
Hal Walter

Cover Design
Kathy Capp

Typography
Out There!

Printed in the United States
Library of Congress Catalog Number: 99-073521
First edition

ISBN 0-9642062-3-4

David Barmore Productions
P.O. Box 250, Todd Road
Stamford, NY 12167

"And ye shall eat the fat of the land."

— Genesis 45:18

"An army marches on its stomach."

— Napoleon Bonaparte

"Give them great meals of beef and iron and steel,
they will eat like wolves and fight like devils."

— William Shakespeare, King Henry V

"Jack Sprat could eat no fat,
His wife could eat no lean;
And so betwixted the both,
They licked the platter clean."

— Jack Sprat, anonymous nursery rhyme

"there is some s. i will not eat"

— ee cummings

"Animals feed themselves, men eat;
but only wise men know the art of eating."

— Anthelme Brillat-Savarin, The Physiology of Taste

"Tell me what you eat,
and I shall tell you what you are."

— Anthelme Brillat-Savarin, The Physiology of Taste

"Choose your food wisely."

— Dr. Phil Maffetone

Table of Contents

Introduction

There is an endless list of components that influence endurance athletic performance. Everything from equipment to mental and spiritual health can make a difference in the outcome of a race. The two elements that can make the most significant difference, however, are the actual workouts that an athete does, and the food that he or she eats.

During my 15-year career as a professional athlete, the attention I gave to diet was critical to my success. Initially what I ate was swayed by the athletic diet *dujour.* Most of the fad perfomance diets were based on bad science that had nothing to do with sustaining performance over time in the real world. Fortunately, I met Dr. Phil Maffetone, who coached me to eat according to what the body actually needs and responds to in training and racing.

The best part of his dietary guidelines is that they followed the balance of my body's natural cravings. There was nothing that went contrary to the voice of my body telling me what to eat. This was very different than my experience with other diets and eating regimens.

The results speak for themselves. I was able to sustain a world-class level in a very demanding endurance sport for 15 years, winning six Ironman Triathlon titles along the way. For anyone interested in reaching peak athletic potential, *Eating for Endurance* is a must. But don't just take my word. Try the guidelines in this book and see the results for yourself!

— ***Mark Allen***

Foreword

I have been following Dr. Phil Maffetone's program since 1991, and the impact it has made on my career as a professional triathlete, and my life in general, has been profound. Now Phil has put all of the ideas about diet and nutrition that he offered as my coach and trainer into one package, *Eating for Endurance.* The ideas Phil presents are off the beaten path and can be found in no other nutrition book on the market. Not only will you find this book helpful in improving athletic performance, it also offers solid ideas for improving health, losing weight and increasing energy.

This information and an open mind are all you need to change your dietary habits. Good health will follow. Over the last century humans have gotten farther and farther from their evolutionary diet. We evolved as hunters and gatherers, but now most people eat more like feedlot cattle. I notice in my own dietary evolution that I began to reach for whole foods rather than processed ones, especially refined carbohydrates. I increased my protein intake by including more meat and eggs. I seriously took stock of my carbohydrate intake, relying mainly on fruit, fresh or steamed vegetables and small amounts of whole grains. I also increased my consumption of healthy fats by adding more avocados, butter, nuts and seeds to my diet. My increased fat and protein intake has given me more energy.

I feel confident promoting Phil's program in my travels and lectures. I'm sure his principles will help you improve your health, build endurance and feel better, whether it's training for the Ironman or just going out and enjoying a hike. *Eating for Endurance* puts all these ideas between two covers.

— ***Mike Pigg***

Preface

In my 20-plus years of working with athletes, the key part of my methodology has been to provide information to help individuals understand how to find the approach that works the best for him or her, as opposed to prescribing a preconceived diet and list of supplements, and inferring all athletes must follow these blindly. I teach each athlete to match his or her specific needs and reap the benefits, which include increased endurance and performance, longer athletic lifespan and significant improvements in overall health, including the elimination of injuries.

This book describes this process.

Here's how you can get the most out of this book. First, understand the basic chapters — those that provide a general overview and philosophy of my eating program. These are outlined in chapters 1-4. You will find this approach very different from most books, diets and nutritional advice. I'm asking that you keep an open mind and take responsibility for your own health and fitness, rather than rely on others to give you the magic pill, which of course does not exist.

Next, understand the basic information on diet and nutrition — general knowledge almost everyone needs to know and follow. This is found in chapters 5-13. These chapters help lay the groundwork that will enable you to more effectively take the necessary steps to individualize your diet and nutrition. Once you get to chapters 14-18, you'll have an easier time individualizing your diet and nutritional state. Chapters 19-24 provide ideas on eating — not just what, but how and when, along with tips how to obtain the highest quality food and get the most out of it. This part also includes a chapter on the next generation of endurance athletes — our children.

Because this is an individualized approach, it is always evolving. It's not a cookbook program you blindly follow without any thought, but rather one that will become your lifestyle. You'll learn to be more intuitive and instinctual regarding eating. As the seasons pass, as your priorities are modified, or as your goals change, you'll be able to easily adjust your diet as necessary to match your unique needs. In the process you may also be able to help family and friends get more healthy and fit.

— *Dr. Phil Maffetone*

1

Nutritional Ergogenics

There are no magic formulas or secret foods that will improve your endurance. But match your body's needs with the appropriate foods, nutrients and natural remedies, and your endurance is likely to improve dramatically. In addition, your body will function optimally, perhaps like it did when you were younger. Or if you're a youngster, you'll avoid the injuries, ill health and poor performances that many athletes experience at alarming rates in their 20s, 30s and later in life. With proper nutrition and training, your endurance could — and should — actually improve well into your 40s.

This book is a companion to my previous work, *Training for Endurance* (David Barmore Productions, 1996). Its aim is to help you find the proper dietary balance that will result in ergogenic nourishment, and ultimately, a higher level of energy and endurance for sports as well as other areas of your life in general.

Ergogenic nourishment refers to the consumption of liquid or solid nutrients to assist in human performance. A balanced diet and nutritional state accomplishes this task to a great extent, and should be the primary focus of your health and fitness program. In addition to a properly matched diet which meets each individual's needs, many athletes also use nutritional ergogenic aids such as sport drinks, gels and energy bars.

Athletes, scientists and clinicians have long agreed that eating habits directly affect endurance. In many cases, it's not a question of the latest research but rather an understanding of basic physiology and biochemistry. For example, it's well known that water is the most important ergogenic aid in sports. Even minor deficiencies can be devastating to your performance results. This same principle applies to electrolytes — a reduced sodium content in the body, for example, will usually have major adverse effects on training and competition.

Let's look at the basic aspect of how we obtain energy for endurance. This simple outline will help you better appreciate food and your body's ability to generate energy from it. It is also the first step in helping you in your quest to find an ideal nutritional program — one which may change from season to season, or year to year, as your body's needs change with training, stress and age.

Energy Production

We all know the human body requires energy to function. But what is the source of this energy, and how does it evolve from its raw source to a fuel for your body?

The true source of your body's energy is the sun. *Light energy* from the sun comes to earth and is converted to *chemical energy* through the process of photosynthesis in plants. This energy is taken into your body when we eat plants, and for most of us, when we eat animals that obtained their energy by eating plants. This chemical energy we take in is then converted to *mechanical energy* which we use to do everything from simple everyday tasks to working out and racing.

In very general terms, our energy is obtained from the foods we eat. These foods contain three macronutrients: carbohydrates, fats and proteins. Though most foods contain all three, there's usually a predominance of one of these macronutrients in most foods. The chart below lists some common examples.

The majority of our energy comes from two of these macronutrients, carbohydrates and fats. A lesser amount of energy is available from protein,

COMMON FOODS HIGH IN SPECIFIC MACRONUTRIENTS		
Carbohydrates	**Fats**	**Proteins**
Bread, sugar, rice, pasta, fruit and fruit juice, cereal	Oils, butter, high-fat cheeses, egg yolk	Meat, fish, poultry, eggs, cheese (curds & whey)

only up to about 15 percent of our total energy. Our bodies convert these macronutrients into energy through two steps. First, they are broken down in the intestine and absorbed into the blood as glucose (from carbohydrates), fatty acids (from fats) and amino acids (from protein). In the second step, the blood takes these elements to the cells, where the molecules of glucose, fatty acids and amino acids are further broken down. The hydrogen atom, the common building block of all three food groups, is released as a result of further chemical breakdown. This atom contains one highly energy-charged electron. This electron is finally converted to a substance called adrenosine triphosphate (ATP), which provides the power we use as energy.

To state it simply, we could say our energy comes from hydrogen's electron. Carbohydrates, fats and proteins all have varying amounts of hydrogen molecules, and therefore potential energy. Fats have by far the most hydrogen, one reason why we can obtain so much more energy from fats. Fats can provide us with more than twice the energy we get from either carbohydrates or proteins. For example, we can get 36 molecules of ATP from a given amount of glucose, and the same amount of fat will yield about 460 molecules of ATP, depending on which particular fat is used. So fat yields nearly 13 times the amount of ATP as glucose.

Harnessing Your Energy

The body has two general "energy systems" which it uses to convert fatty acids and carbohydrates into energy. These are the aerobic and anaerobic systems. In each individual these systems have both structural and chemical aspects. They generate energy from specific substrates — fatty acids and glucose — to produce movement.

Where does all this energy-generating activity take place? Mostly it is created by our metabolism in the aerobic muscle fibers, with some occurring in anaerobic fibers. When these fibers are functioning optimally, you can derive even more energy from fats — up to 80 percent at any given time — with the remainder coming from carbohydrates. This high amount of "fat-burning" is possible at rest. As activity intensifies, more carbohydrate and less fat is burned. At moderate levels of training, a good amount of fat can be burned, depending upon the nutrient content of your previous meal (the amounts of carbohydrates and fats), and how you've programmed your metabolism through training (how well your aerobic muscle fibers function).

In order for these raw materials (glucose and fat) to be burned for energy, certain micronutrients are necessary. Some of these include a number of the B vitamins (thiamin, riboflavin, pyridoxine and niacin), and certain minerals like magnesium, manganese and iron. This issue is addressed later.

Fact: many athletes do not consume enough of these nutrients in their daily diet.

Dietary fat usually goes into storage after being absorbed by the body. The stored fat we all have also represents a tremendous reserve of potential energy. A lean athlete can store up to 100,000 kilocalories of energy from fat, but glucose stores are nowhere near as great. This contrast is put into clinical perspective by Newsholm (1977):

The energy reserves from fat in a healthy athlete can power a run for 119 hours, with reserves from glucose allowing the energy for only a 1.6-hour run.

During rest, fat may contribute significant amounts of energy, up to 60-80 percent, or more. The same is true during light to moderate workouts, where fat may provide 50 percent (or more in athletes with great aerobic function) of the necessary energy. During longer training periods and competitions, much higher percentages may be available from fats — up to 80 percent or more. From a standpoint of athletic performance, Lambert et al. (1994) and Muoio (1994) demonstrated improvements in performance following a *higher*-fat diet, which made more fat available for energy. And Vukovich (1993) showed that an increased consumption of dietary fat spared stored glycogen during exercise, an important function for endurance and competition.

To maintain efficient fat-burning, we also must burn some sugar. Both fat and sugar are almost always being burned for energy at all times. Right now, you may be getting half of your energy from fat and half from sugar. When you improve your aerobic system and fat-burning capabilities, you may be able to obtain 70 percent of your energy from fat and 30 percent from sugar. But many people can only get 10 percent of their energy from fat, forcing a full 90 percent to come from sugar. That's a very inefficient way to get energy, and it could lead to fatigue, increased body-fat stores (sugar not capable of being immediately used for energy — roughly 40 percent or more — is stored as fat), and other problems discussed throughout this book.

Measuring Fat and Sugar Burning

This mix of fuels can be easily measured in a person with a gas analyzer, which measures the amount of oxygen a person takes into his or her body and the amount of carbon dioxide eliminated. The ratio of carbon dioxide to oxygen is called the respiratory quotient (RQ), and from it is determined the percentage of fat and sugar used for energy. From my experience in more than 20 years of private practice, I have found that a lower RQ corresponds to greater fat-burning and a higher level of aerobic fitness. I do not recommend most people have an RQ test because it can be difficult to find a doctor with the equipment to administer this test and the test can be expensive. However, it is useful for you to understand the RQ concept is order to better understand the physiology of how my program will improve your endurance.

The normal range of RQ is from 0.7 to 1.0. In this range, 0.7 is 100 percent fat-burning and 0 percent sugar burning; at the other end of the continuum 1.0 represents 0 percent fat-burning and 100 percent sugar burning. Neither of these extremes usually happens in real life. Rather, the body usually uses a mix of these fuels. For example, an RQ of 0.85 is a mix of about 50 percent fat and 50 percent sugar burning; an RQ of 0.91 is a mix of about 30 percent fat and 70 percent sugar, and an RQ of 0.79 is about 70 percent fat and 30 percent sugar. So, the lower the RQ in a person, the higher that person's fat-burning capability.

Measuring a person's RQ on a stationary bike or treadmill enables us to see how the amounts of fat and sugar used to produce energy change with intensity. As noted above, the higher the physical intensity (i.e., the heart rate), the more sugar and less fat is burned; this is seen in the test in the form of a higher RQ. The right training promotes higher amounts of fat-burning at higher levels of intensity. Over time, this will enable an athlete to develop more speed at a lower heart rate — maintaining a level of intensity at which the body is still deriving much of its energy from fat. So, as your body becomes capable of burning more fat as its primary fuel, your energy becomes greater, and your endurance and speed will increase. In addition, it's common to see better health associated with improved utilization of fat as a fuel. Following is a list of some patient's RQ numbers at rest and their symptoms. Take away the patient initials and the chart could really be one person who progresses on my program. In general, the less sugar and more fat-burning at any level of intensity, the more healthy and fit the individual.

NAME	RQ AS % SUGAR AND FAT	COMPLAINTS
JC	88% sugar, 12% fat	extreme fatigue, insomnia, 45 pounds overweight
BK	74% sugar, 26% fat	afternoon & evening fatigue, asthma, headaches
JO	62% sugar, 38% fat	afternoon fatigue, seasonal allergies, 10 pounds overweight
PS	55% sugar, 45% fat	chronic, mild knee pain, indigestion
MK	42% sugar, 58% fat	occasional low-back pain
BE	37% sugar, 63% fat	none

Eating Food vs. Absorbing Nutrients

Eating the right foods may provide us with the glucose (from carbohydrates), fatty acids (from fats), amino acids (from protein), and all the necessary vitamins and minerals to generate significant amounts of energy. However, just eating the right foods does not guarantee your body will assimilate those vital substances, or absorb them in the right proportions. There are four important steps required for your body to benefit from food.

The most important aspect of diet is its quality. If we choose to consume too much processed food, we risk obtaining too little of the micronutrients necessary to make energy for endurance. For example, processed grains, as opposed to whole-grain products (a bagel instead of 100-percent whole-grain bread, for instance), often lack certain nutrients such as thiamin (vitamin B1). An inadequate amount of this nutrient could adversely affect energy production and the ability to break down lactic acid, another important bodily function. Eating real foods, and avoiding processed items is the first step to getting more energy for endurance. The list below contains just some examples of real foods which should be substituted for processed foods. It's important to read the labels on the food products which state the type of food they contain. Most real foods either don't have a list of ingredients, or the list is real short, naming just the real foods contained. In addition, if an ingredient is difficult to pronounce, it's probably not real food.

In the case of real versus processed foods, both choices are easily available, and the cost factor is not a significant issue (it's actually cheaper to eat foods of higher quality, especially when you consider the health benefits).

Digestion is the second step necessary to obtain the benefits of food. Once you eat a meal, the food undergoes a long and complex process of digestion. If this process is efficient, more nutrients will be available for use by your body.

The first stage of digestion is activity in the brain and nervous system. If we are stressed (angry, rushing, working, training), our ability to effi-

EXAMPLES OF PROCESSED FOODS	VS. REAL FOOD OPTIONS
Rolls, bagels, most breads (including those labeled wheat flour), most crackers, puffed products and processed cereals (except oats, shredded wheat and wheat germ).	100% whole-wheat bread, crackers and cereals.
White rice	Brown rice
Fats and oils: all hydrogenated and partially hydrogenated oils, tropical oils (palm and palm kernel), all fractionated oils.	Extra-virgin olive oil
Limit or avoid all polyunsaturated oils as they are chemically unstable. These include: safflower, sunflower, corn, soybean.	Extra-virgin olive oil
Processed protein items: soy isolates, protein caseinates, textured protein, hydrolyzed protein*	Unprocessed protein sources: whey, egg-white powder, soy powder, soy beans

** Though not listed as an ingredient, all isolates, caseinates (a milk protein), and hydrolyzed proteins also contain monosodium glutamate (MSG) as a by-product of processing these proteins.*

ciently digest food is impaired, and proper digestion may not take place. It is important to plan your meals so that you are in a relaxed state. A prayer before meals, a glass of wine or sitting down with people you want to be with are all examples of ways to help prepare your body to relax and digest your meal. In addition, listening to enjoyable music can also help with digestion because of its stress-reducing capabilities.

The first physical stage of digestion is in the mouth. Here several factors begin the digestive process. The teeth are important to chop food into smaller pieces to increase efficiency of chemical digestion lower in the digestive tract. It's important to chew your food well. However, I don't urge people to count how many times they chew their food as this can be stressful. Just be aware that chewing each mouthful completely is very important. Those with dental problems often have difficulty chewing food properly, and may have significant digestion problems as a result. If you have dental problems it is imperative to seek proper care to correct them.

There are also a variety of enzymes in the saliva which start the chemical aspect of digestion in the mouth. This is especially important in the digestion of carbohydrates. Be sure to chew your breads, rice, legumes, fruits and other carbohydrate foods well. Certain chemicals in the mouth also affect the breakdown of fats.

From the mouth, food is swallowed into the stomach. The two most important aspects of digestion here are the mixing of food, and the chemical action of hydrochloric acid. Food is mixed in the stomach by the three layers of muscle which make up the stomach. This is the reason you may feel and hear noises from your upper abdomen — there's a lot of churning going on there, especially after a meal.

Hydrochloric acid normally is secreted when food enters the stomach, and is vital to good digestion. This natural acid stimulates other digestive enzymes, especially for the breakdown of protein. Hydrochloric acid also chemically changes various dietary substances such as calcium, and kills bacteria, viruses and other potentially harmful invaders which enter through almost all foods. Reducing your hydrochloric acid with antacids following a meal can be detrimental. Protein digestion may be impaired, and you may not absorb the much-needed amino acids. This can also trigger immune-system reactions if undigested (whole proteins) are absorbed. This is one cause of allergies. Inadequate levels of hydrochloric acid can cause vitamin and mineral deficiencies, since without proper digestion of food, these nutrients are not available for absorption. Also, the potential for bacterial, yeast and fungal infections is high when hydrochloric acid levels are reduced. In addition, without the hydrochloric acid effect on such things as calcium (which changes to a more readily absorbable form), calcium absorption may be significantly diminished.

Taking antacids is not the only thing that will reduce levels of hydrochloric acid. Normal aging often results in lower levels, as does any type of stress. (Note that *some* people under stress have hydrochloric-acid production when the stomach is empty — a time when this should not happen.) Drinking large amounts of liquids with meals may also dilute stomach acid and enzymes resulting in less-efficient digestion.

During my years in practice, it was not unusual to recommend supplements such as betaine hydrochloride (which turns to hydrochloric acid) for people who did not produce enough of their own acid. Common symptoms in these individuals included belching and bloating after a protein meal, bad breath, loss of appetite (especially for meat), and large amounts of foul-smelling gas.

Hydrochloric acid also triggers action and further digestion in the small intestine, including secretion of proteolytic enzymes from the pancreas. Following this stage, digestion should be complete and your body ready to reap the benefits.

Once nutrients are made available through the action of digestion, they can now undergo the action of absorption into the body. (Note that once inside the intestine, foods are not yet "in" the body but outside the body. It's much like being in the hole of a doughnut.) The process of nutritional absorption is the third key step in getting nutrients out of your diet. The small intestine, with its finger-like projections called villi, are capable of pulling nutrients from the now well-digested foods. Certain portions of the small intestine absorb specific nutrients as they pass, and the nutrients enter the blood.

The function of the villi is vital for good nutrient absorption. Stress, poor digestion and not eating (dieting, fasting, hospitalization) can significantly impair absorption. In addition, the villi use an important amino acid, L-glutamine, to obtain the energy required for the absorptive mechanism. Without adequate glutamine, absorption of nutrients can also be impaired.

Once nutrients are absorbed into the body, they complete their fourth step, utilization. Once into the blood, nutrients are carried to the liver for processing. The liver acts like a manufacturing plant and distribution center. Some nutrients rely on others for their utilization. For example, calcium must rely on certain essential fats to be utilized or carried into a bone or muscle for final use. Other nutrients, such as thiamin, can go directly into cells to help generate energy for endurance.

The macronutrients are also utilized quickly after absorption. Glucose is acted upon by insulin and used for energy, stored as fat, or stored as glycogen. Fats are sent to muscles for use as energy, with some going to storage. Amino acids are used in many different ways. They help in many aspects of metabolism and cell repair, and small amounts also are used for energy.

The whole spectrum of generating energy for endurance is a long and complex process. With increased efficiency, more energy can be gained. Much of this action can be improved by you deciding to improve your energy-generating potential by choosing high-quality foods, eating in a relaxed environment and not tampering with your body's natural digestive mechanism.

2

Individualizing Your Diet

Everyone is familiar with dieting. It is the subject of weekly tabloids, television talk shows and *New York Times* best-sellers. There are diets for everything, but nowhere is the concept of dieting more misused and misunderstood than in the field of sports nutrition. The most popular diets prescribed for athletes are those high in carbohydrates.

The approach I have taken in my work with athletes of all abilities is that each person has unique dietary requirements, and my job is to help the athlete find his or her proper *balance* of carbohydrates, proteins and fats. This process involves an understanding of how the body works, following true instincts of diet selection, and avoiding the marketing hype so prevalent in the sports community. Other methods of dieting — such as following a general menu rather than an individualized approach — are not as effective. Some of these, the common calorie-counting approach and the 40-30-30 diet for instance, are discussed below. It should also be mentioned that the quantity of food necessary for athletes also varies with each individual. Studies show that daily diets of elite athletes vary from 1,865 kilocalories to more than 6,000 kilocalories. And percentages of energy macronutrients also range dramatically.

Following Your Instincts

Dietary self-selection is a topic of controversy, although many scientific studies, mostly from animals, demonstrate its existence. In 1928, Clara Davis was one of the first to show the intuitive and instinctual aspects of self-selection of foods in human infants, and published her studies in scientific journals. Other researchers have shown various self-selection in animals. These include self-selection between high- and low-protein diets and diets to maintain acid-alkaline balance. It was demonstrated that animals who are free to self-select their foods ate more fat *but* lost more body fat than those on regular feedings.

In recent years, scientists have learned more about the possible mechanisms of intuitive self-selection. This may involve the liver, nervous system and areas of the brain called the hypothalmus. While developing your instincts, there are a number of ways to help find your ideal diet. Consider these factors:

- The act of writing down your weekly diet *as meals are eaten* rather than on recall (i.e., recalling all the food eaten over the past day or week) can have a significant impact. Following this exercise, many people report they were unaware of how much (or little) they consume, how poorly they eat, or other factors regarding their eating habits.
- Become more aware of any important relationships between your stress and diet. For example, intestinal discomfort occurring during a morning workout following breakfast compared to feeling good following a mid-afternoon workout three hours after lunch; or having a bad workout when a sugared drink is consumed before training.
- Don't hesitate to do your own food "trials," such as a preworkout meal, experimenting with drinks or solid food during a long bike ride, or monitoring the effects of a certain evening meal when your workout is first thing in the morning.
- Always know that your needs may be unique and often significantly different than those of your training companions. And, these needs may change with time of year, training and competition, and aging. So once you find your ideal diet, it soon may change a bit.
- Consider subjecting your diet to a computerized analysis, which is discussed in the next chapter. This takes the guesswork out of your diet's quality.

For some athletes, even thinking about diet causes stress, and occasionally leads to more serious problems. Eating disorders are common in athletes, especially women, and often involve reduced intake of appropriate kilocalories in relation to energy expenditure. Female athletes have an incidence of eating disorders as high as 62 percent. This is a complex issue with a full spectrum of eating problems from functional to pathological disorders, from poor eating habits, dieting and preoccupation with low-fat eating habits, at one end of the continuum, to anorexia nervosa and bulimia at the other. Menstrual problems are frequently associated with eating disorders at all ranges of this spectrum, and with overtraining. Menstrual problems are twice as high in female runners who are vegetarians as compared to those who eat meat. If you have menstrual problems, it means something is not right, and it's important to seek help from a professional who can consider all aspects of your life — from sports and diet to hormones, psychology and stress.

There are varying opinions regarding an ideal diet. Some traditional suggestions include a predominant carbohydrate diet of 60 to 70 percent, with 12 to 15 percent from protein and the remainder from fat. Others have shown that these high-carbohydrate intakes may not provide additional performance benefits (which is the inaccurate reason many athletes follow these diets in the first place). According to some experts, many athletes follow high-carbohydrate, low-fat diets out of fear of eating too much fat and protein. The current U.S. Food Guide Pyramid suggests, for a 2,800 kcal diet, 55 percent carbohydrate, 30 percent fat and 15 percent protein. A discussion about the food pyramid is found in Chapter 4.

The Calorie Counters

The calorie-counting theory says that the calories in the food you eat, minus the calories you burn for energy, equals your weight gain or loss. If you eat fewer calories than you burn, you lose weight. But if you take in more than you use, you gain. And, balancing energy intake and output results in stable weight. The problem with this theory is that it does not work as easily or as frequently as the diet books and businesses indicate. The reason is that everyone has a different metabolism, so food is utilized differently, and fat and sugar are burned at different ratios from person to person. For example, some people get 60 percent of their energy from fat and 40 percent from sugar, where others are just the opposite. In addition to the number of calories taken in, the amount of carbohydrates, fats and proteins eaten also significantly affects how the body burns energy. So to use only the total calories as a guide is highly inaccurate. In addition, calorie counting does not consider where those calories come from, the quality of food, or the balance of macronutrients. More importantly, counting calories doesn't really work in real life. Even worse are the side effects that dieting often creates; the least damaging being weight gain.

Case History

When Sally turned 30, she decided to get serious about dropping the excess weight. So she followed a low-fat diet that limited her caloric intake to 1,000 per day. Within three months, Sally felt more tired, but finally reached her goal of losing 20 pounds. Within six months, she gained about 25 pounds back. She went back on her diet, and it was just as successful as before, although it took a little longer to lose the 25 pounds. This vicious cycle continued for about five years. Sally was now not only tired, but depressed, and suffered from insomnia in addition to PMS for two weeks each month.

During my initial consultation with Sally, I explained how she was continually suppressing her metabolism and getting more unhealthy with each vicious cycle. Sally was weaned off her calorie counting and eventually was able to eat as much as her body required. She eventually got down to the same size clothes she wore when she was at her ideal "weight" at 22 years of age. And to her surprise, the number of calories she was eating was about 2,000 each day!

Calorie counting almost always results in eating less food. When you eat less food, especially less fat which contains the most calories, one of the significant results can be that your metabolism slows down and you can eventually store more fat, despite your initial (short-term) weight loss. That's why so many people eventually gain more fat after being on a calorie-restricted diet. The best way to speed up metabolism is to eat the amount of good quality food you need each day. (Other factors that increase the metabolism are dietary fats and aerobic exercise.)

Knowing the weight in grams of each food eaten at a meal can have more practical meaning than knowing the calories of that meal. Counting grams at least considers all the macronutrients individually. The best example is knowing how many grams of carbohydrate there are in a given food or meal. Along with other factors, this measurement has an important relationship with the amount of insulin produced by the pancreas.

But counting grams can also maintain the dieting obsession. Each time you eat something you have to think about how much it weighs or you have to look it up in a food table. Most people eventually get tired of doing that and fall off their "diet."

The 40-30-30 Myth

This diet's plan is that you eat 40 percent of your calories from carbohydrate, 30 percent from protein and 30 percent from fat. By doing this, the production of insulin is moderated and fat-burning is improved. Unfortunately, you are still left to count calories, maintaining that potential obsession. The real problem is that even if you do eat a 40-30-30 meal, there is no guarantee that your intestines will absorb that same ratio; chances are they won't. Since this diet works by affecting your metabolism, putting the food into your stomach does not yet have a complete effect on your metabolism. Only after absorption from the intestines does that happen.

There are three important factors which can change the ratio of your 40-30-30 meal. These factors all relate to digestion and absorption. One has to do with the amount of usable versus unusable carbohydrates in your food. Another is protein's ability to efficiently digest into amino acids, and third is the fact that some of the fatty acids in food fats don't absorb well. Any or all of these factors can significantly change the 40-30-30 ratio into something different.

Many carbohydrate foods contain fiber. Real, whole food contains higher amounts of natural fiber, but processed foods are often very low or void of fiber. Since fiber is not absorbed into the body, its caloric value can not be considered. When counting grams of carbohydrates, for example, the total equals the difference between the total grams of carbohydrate and the grams of fiber. So if your diet has 40 percent carbohydrate, you're probably including the amount in fiber, which is a misrepresentation.

Protein digestibility is another important factor in the 40-30-30 diet. The efficiency of protein digestion is very much related to your level of stress. The more stress you have, the less effectively you can digest protein food into its components, amino acids. And unless you digest protein into amino acids, it cannot be absorbed. So eating a 40-30-30 meal if you're stressed can result in absorbing much less of the protein you eat.

The issue of fats is different. Fats are made up of many different components called fatty acids. Some of these fatty acids, such as arachidic acid, are not well absorbed under any circumstance. The result? Your fat intake is probably not the same as the amount you absorb and therefore the amount that stimulates your metabolism.

If all this sounds too complicated, you're right. Why count calories or grams? Why blindly follow some menu when you can do what the animals do — eat when you're hungry, eat what you feel your body needs, and stop when you're satisfied? As simple and natural as this sounds, however, you may need some education and practice to reap the benefits. But once you develop your instincts, you'll be free from the obsessions and life — at least from an eating standpoint — will be much more simple.

For many individuals, the first step in this healthy process is evaluating your ability to tolerate carbohydrates. Here's an easy test to see if further assessment is necessary. Answer these questions:

- ❑ Are you frequently or always hungry?
- ❑ Are you irritable or weak before meals or if meals are skipped?
- ❑ Do you frequently crave sweets?
- ❑ Do you often have feeling of depression, or are depressed?
- ❑ Do you get sleepy or experience reduced mental concentration following meals?
- ❑ Do you have intestinal bloating (gas) following meals?
- ❑ Does overeating carbohydrates or sweets make you feel bad?
- ❑ Do you avoid eating breakfast because it increases hunger during the day?
- ❑ Do the above symptoms improve with increased number of meals (i.e., five or six daily meals instead of two or three)?
- ❑ Do you have a history of oral contraceptive use?

If you answered "yes" to three or more of these questions, you should consider taking the Two-Week Test described in Chapter 14. These questions, and the symptoms they describe, are often associated with an excess intake of carbohydrates, especially the refined types. This test will help you determine how much carbohydrate is best for your body. Once you determine that, you're on your way to finding your ideal diet.

The first step in finding your optimal eating plan is to assses your current diet, including how much you're really eating, the ratio of carbohydrate, fat and protein, the status of your vitamins and minerals and other important aspects of your diet.

3

Analyzing Your Diet

An early step in improving your energy for endurance is evaluating your diet. Does it contain all the macro- and micronutrients necessary to give you unlimited energy for endurance? Most people are not sure. Those who think they know what they are eating usually are surprised at their actual dietary analysis. In general, most people are aghast at the nutritional content of their diets.

Your dietary habits, assuming they've been somewhat consistent, can give you an objective idea of your nutritional status. For example, if your diet is low in magnesium and vitamin B6 (two common nutritional insufficiencies), there is a good chance that your body is too low in these essential nutrients. Unless you supplement your diet with both nutrients, you may remain low for a long time, even if your new diet has sufficient amounts. In other words, it could take a long time to correct a nutritional imbalance by eating the right foods, but that same nutritional problem could be corrected much quicker with supplementation (discussed in later chapters). Once you've made some healthy changes to your diet you'll also want to have your new diet analyzed for nutritional content.

This book addresses nutrition from a functional standpoint, rather than from the perspective of disease and preventing deficiency diseases which are rare in industrialized countries. Research has shown that your body may require specific nutrients to improve physical, chemical and mental/emotional function, even when blood tests are normal for these nutrients. Many people fall into the gap between overt deficiency and the levels of nutrient intake that allow optimal function, such as increased energy for endurance.

Recommendations used in this book, and by the companies which perform computerized analyses, do not necessarily agree with the recommended dietary allowances (RDAs) which are mostly disease-based. For example, the RDA for vitamin C is 60 mg/day for adults. The U.S. Food and Nutrition Board says this dose is based on preventing signs and symptoms of scurvy for at least four weeks if there is no vitamin C intake. In addition, the RDA is designed explicitly to be applicable to populations rather than to individuals. However, the use of RDA values may have some benefit in that it can serve as a general guide when comparing your "old" and "new" diets.

Unfortunately, the intakes of some individuals do not even meet these RDA levels for some nutrients. This may especially be true in athletes who are restricting energy intake to achieve weight loss, and those involved in competition. In fact, weight loss by energy restriction reduces competitive ability.

How to Analyze Your Diet

The best and most practical way to assess your diet is by computer. This can be accomplished with three different options. There are a number of diet programs you can purchase for your own computer. These usually print out some type of report highlighting the amounts of certain nutrients. Your doctor or other health-care professional may be able to provide this service for you. The third approach is to go directly to a company which performs this service. NutrAnalysis, Inc., is one such company that offers dietary analysis, including an extensive 14-page report for your records.

An alternative to using a computer program or hiring a dietary-analysis service is to look up each food in a book which gives the amounts of each nutrient and add them all up. This is very tedious and could take days to complete. Considering that you'll also want to check your newly modified and improved diet based on the recommendations in this book and other information, and probably experiment on paper to see which foods added or removed give the best outcome for your needs, using a computer's capability makes the most sense. Whatever approach you choose, it is vital that a complete assessment is performed. This is described below.

What to Measure in Your Diet

It's definitely worth the effort to evaluate your diet. But if you take the time, and put forth the effort and expense to evaluate your dietary habits, be sure to do so in as effective and complete a manner as possible. Be sure that at least the following items are evaluated when performing this analysis:

- ❑ Total calories
- ❑ Percent carbohydrate, protein and fat
- ❑ Vitamin and mineral levels
- ❑ Amino-acid levels
- ❑ Essential fatty-acid levels
- ❑ Omega-3 and omega-6 fat ratio
- ❑ Percentages of monounsaturated, polyunsaturated and saturated fat
- ❑ Amount of fiber

In addition to these items, a written report should be given for your records. Below are some sample pages from the NutrAnalysis report. Note that some of the charts list such items as "Nutrients needed for energy production" and "Nutrients needed for antioxidant activity." If the report is very complete, you should not need a professional's interpretation.

After Your Diet Assessment

Once you know what nutrients, if any, are too low in your diet, you'll need to do two things. First, it's important to know what foods you need to eat

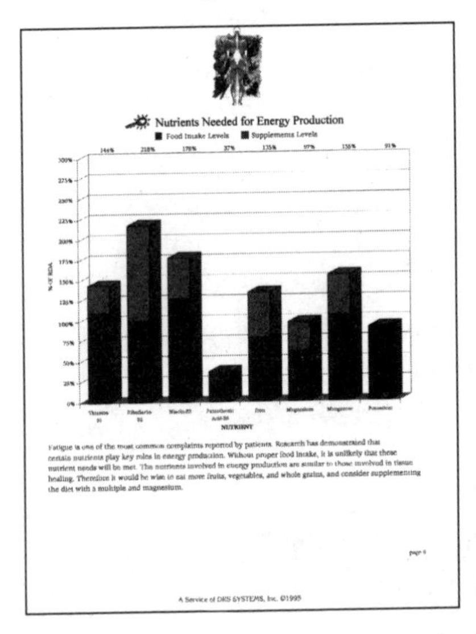

Fatigue is one of the most common complaints reported by patients. Research has demonstrated that certain nutrients play key roles in energy production. Without proper food intake, it is unlikely that these nutrient needs will be met. The nutrients involved in energy production are similar to those involved in tissue healing. Therefore it would be wise to eat more fruits, vegetables, and whole grains, and consider supplementing the diet with a multiple and magnesium.

A Service of DRS SYSTEMS, Inc. ©1995

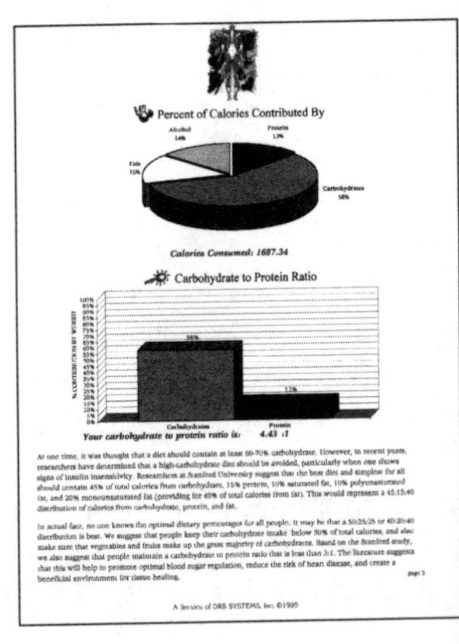

At one time, it was thought that a diet should contain at least 60-70% carbohydrate. However, in recent years, researchers have determined that a high-carbohydrate diet should be avoided, particularly when one shows signs of insulin insensitivity. Researchers at Stanford University suggest that the best diet and simplest for all should contain 45% of total calories from carbohydrate, 15% protein, 10% saturated fat, 10% polyunsaturated fat, and 20% monounsaturated fat (providing for 40% of total calories from fat). This would represent a 45:15:40 distribution of calories from carbohydrate, protein, and fat.

In actual fact, no one knows the optimal dietary percentages for all people. It may be that a 50:25:25 or 40:20:40 distribution is best. We suggest that people keep their carbohydrate intake below 50% of total calories, and also make sure that vegetables and fruits make up the great majority of carbohydrates. Based on the Stanford study, we also suggest that people maintain a carbohydrate to protein ratio that is less than 3:1. The literature suggests that this will help to promote optimal blood sugar regulation, reduce the risk of heart disease, and create a beneficial environment for tissue healing.

page 3

A Service of DRS SYSTEMS, Inc. ©1995

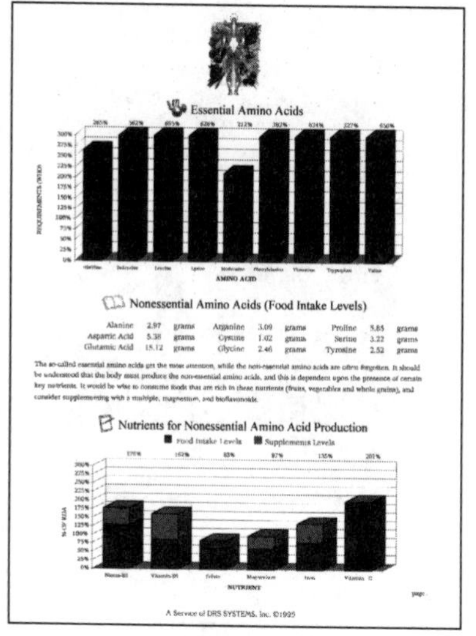

Essential Amino Acids

AMINO ACID

Nonessential Amino Acids (Food Intake Levels)

Alanine	2.97	grams	Arganine	3.09	grams	Proline	5.85	grams
Aspartic Acid	5.38	grams	Cystine	1.02	grams	Serine	3.22	grams
Glutamic Acid	15.12	grams	Glycine	2.46	grams	Tyrosine	2.52	grams

The so-called essential amino acids get the most attention, while the non-essential amino acids are often forgotten. It should be understood that the body must produce the non-essential amino acids, and this is dependent upon the presence of certain key nutrients. It would be wise to consume foods that are rich in these nutrients (fruits, vegetables and whole grains), and consider supplementing with a multiple, magnesium, and bioflavonoids.

Nutrients for Nonessential Amino Acid Production

Food Intake Levels Supplements Levels

NUTRIENT

A Service of DRS SYSTEMS, Inc. ©1995

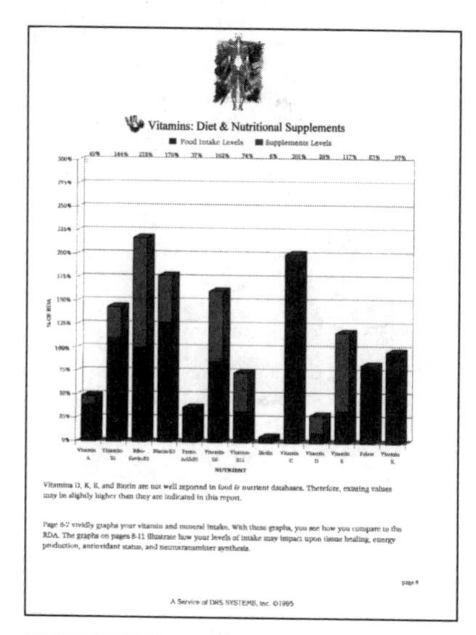

Vitamins: Diet & Nutritional Supplements

Food Intake Levels Supplements Levels

NUTRIENT

Vitamins D, K, E, and Biotin are not well reported in food & nutrient databases. Therefore, existing values may be slightly higher than they are indicated in this report.

Page 6-7 vividly graphs your vitamin and mineral intake. With these graphs, you see how you compare to the RDA. The graphs on pages 8-11 illustrate how your levels of intake may impact upon tissue healing, energy production, antioxidant status, and neurotransmitter synthesis.

page 6

A Service of DRS SYSTEMS, Inc. ©1995

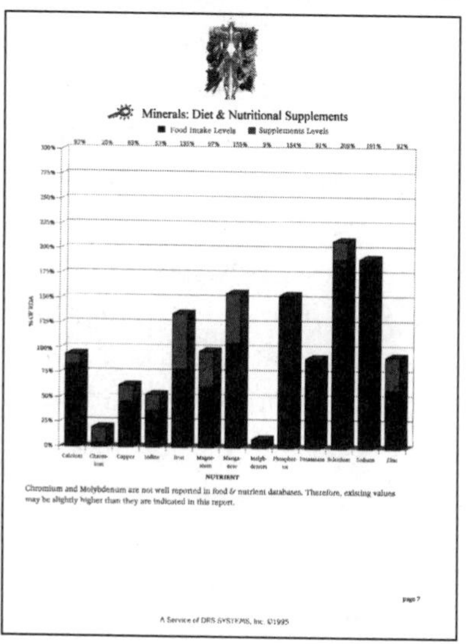

Minerals: Diet & Nutritional Supplements

Food Intake Levels Supplements Levels

NUTRIENT

Chromium and Molybdenum are not well reported in food & nutrient databases. Therefore, existing values may be slightly higher than they are indicated in this report.

page 7

A Service of DRS SYSTEMS, Inc. ©1995

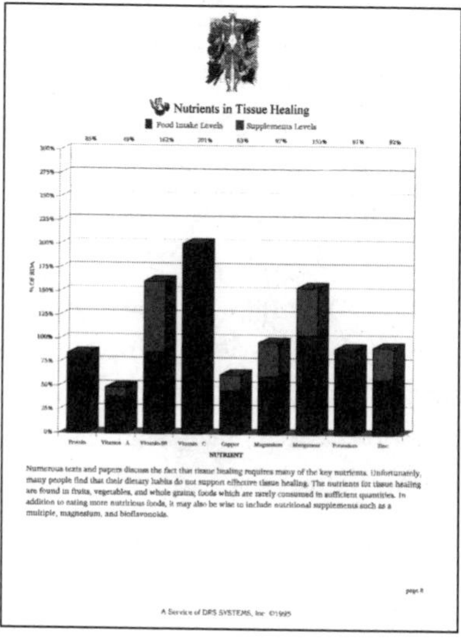

Nutrients in Tissue Healing

Food Intake Levels Supplements Levels

NUTRIENT

Numerous texts and papers discuss the fact that tissue healing requires many of the key nutrients. Unfortunately, many people find that their dietary habits do not support effective tissue healing. The nutrients for tissue healing are found in fruits, vegetables, and whole grains; foods which are rarely consumed in sufficient quantities. In addition to eating more nutritious foods, it may also be wise to include nutritional supplements such as a multiple, magnesium, and bioflavonoids.

page 8

A Service of DRS SYSTEMS, Inc. ©1995

more of to restore normal nutrient levels. A good report should tell you this.

Most importantly, it has always been my practice to supplement an individual with that nutrient for a short period of time (typically about three to four months) to immediately restore the body's levels. If you don't, can't or won't eat foods high in the nutrients you are lacking, you should consider taking the associated supplement indefinitely, since you have no other way of supplying your body with that nutrient.

In addition, after your initial dietary analysis (and after reading chapters

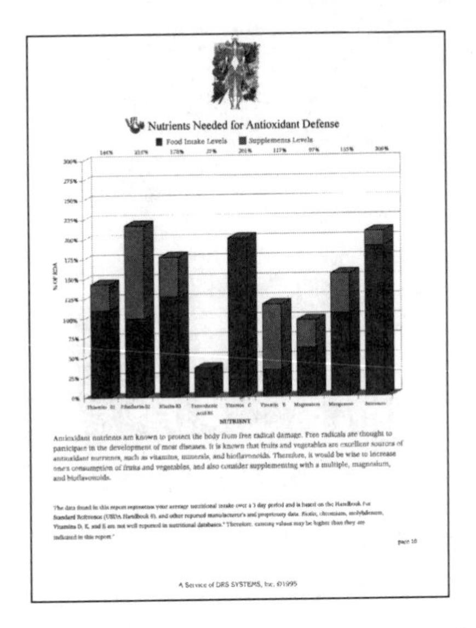

Nutrients Needed for Antioxidant Defense

Food Intake Levels Supplements Levels

NUTRIENT

Antioxidant nutrients are known to protect the body from free radical damage. Free radicals are thought to participate in the development of most diseases. It is known that fruits and vegetables are excellent sources of antioxidant nutrients, such as vitamins, minerals, and bioflavonoids. Therefore, it would be wise to increase one's consumption of fruits and vegetables, and also consider supplementing with a multiple, magnesium, and bioflavonoids.

page 10

A Service of DRS SYSTEMS, Inc. ©1995

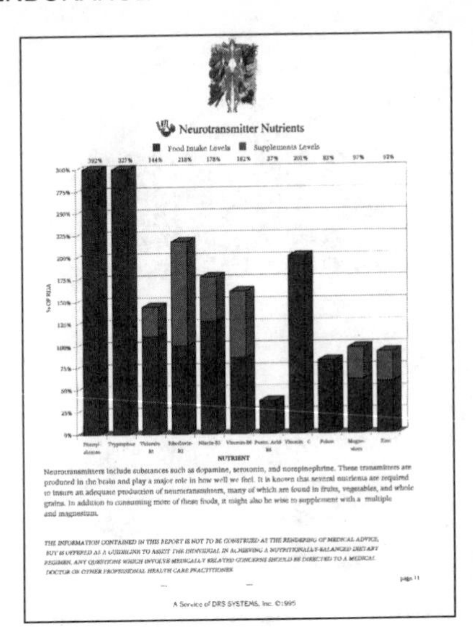

Neurotransmitter Nutrients

Food Intake Levels Supplements Levels

NUTRIENT

Neurotransmitters include substances such as dopamine, serotonin, and norepinephrine. These transmitters are produced in the brain and play a major role in how well we feel. It is known that several nutrients are required to insure an adequate production of neurotransmitters, many of which are found in fruits, vegetables, and whole grains. In addition to consuming more of these foods, it might also be wise to supplement with a multiple and magnesium.

THE INFORMATION CONTAINED IN THIS REPORT IS NOT TO BE CONSTRUED AS THE RENDERING OF MEDICAL ADVICE, BUT IS OFFERED AS A GUIDELINE TO ASSIST THE INDIVIDUAL IN ACHIEVING A NUTRITIONALLY-BALANCED DIETARY REGIMEN. ANY QUESTIONS WHICH INVOLVE MEDICALLY RELATED CONCERNS SHOULD BE DIRECTED TO A MEDICAL DOCTOR OR OTHER PROFESSIONAL HEALTH CARE PRACTITIONER.

page 11

A Service of DRS SYSTEMS, Inc. ©1995

2 and 3), you may make some significant changes in your diet. This may be modifying macronutrient content (changing carbohydrate, fat and protein ratios), increasing more foods specific to your nutritional needs, or reducing certain foods that cause an imbalance in fats (i.e., too much omega-6 oil, for example). Once you have established a good eating routine, which could take several weeks or months, it's a good idea to re-evaluate your diet.

Re-evaluating your diet will ensure that your "new" eating program is providing you with the optimal intake of nutrients. It will also check to make sure you have improved on the intake of nutrients which were previously too low. It makes almost no sense to evaluate your diet the first time without a recheck.

4

The Pyramid Scheme

In 1992 the United States Department of Agriculture (USDA) decided its dietary guideline program known as the "four food groups" (there were really five) was not enough, and created the Food Pyramid. Ironically, this pyramid stands today as a figurative monument over an overweight and disease-ridden society.

You too can make your own food pyramid! Actually, that's the only sound recommendation. Since we all have individual requirements, it's best for each of us to have an individualized pyramid.

As with much that comes out of our nation's capital, there are a number of problems associated with this "pyramid scheme." If it had been truly created by a team of scientists and clinicians with the aim of making general health recommendations, it may have turned out well. However, it was as much a lobbying effort as anything else. Special-interest groups from the food industry had their input, with the result being a misguided public-information program. Unfortunately these lobbysists and their puppets who set policies were thinking of the pyramid on the back of the dollar bill rather than a helpful guide for nutrition.

Disappointed with this nutritional misguidance, some groups have made their own pyramid. Assisted by the Harvard School of Public Health, some of these pyramids are alternatives to what is called the outdated U.S. government Food Guide Pyramid, which has done little to stem the tide of weight gain and health problems facing Americans. For more information, check www.oldwayspt.org/html/pyramid.html on the Internet.

Edward Siguel, M.D., Ph.D., in his letter published in the September 1995 issue of the *American Journal of Clinical Nutrition*, states, "The USDA alleges that the Food Pyramid reflects up-to-date knowledge of nutrition. However, the implicit and explicit assumptions/citations in the USDA's Pyramid justification are scientifically incorrect, as they are based on obsolete recommendations." Specific problems with the current USDA Pyramid include imbalances of essential fatty acids, high-glycemic carbohydrate excess and low nutrient levels.

Essential Fatty Acid Imbalance

As previously discussed, certain fats in our diet are essential for good health. These are termed essential fatty acids (EFAs) and include omega-6 and omega-3 found in certain oils. These fats are consumed in such foods as vegetables, fish and especially oils like flaxseed (linseed); supplement forms include black currant seed oil and EPA (fish oil). However, the current pyramid has fats at the very top and recommends that fats be used sparingly. The importance of EFA balance is not even mentioned in the USDA guidelines.

Siguel further states: "For example, a slim woman eating 1,500 kcal/day who faithfully follows the USDA Food Pyramid easily obtains 700 calories from breads, pasta and cereals. The remaining 800 calories may come from vegetables, fruits, chicken and low-fat dairy products. From these foods she cannot possibly get (the required) 15-20 grams of (omega-6 and omega-3) EFAs/day."

Siguel estimates that in the United States, EFA imbalance affects more than 50 million people. If people actually follow the pyramid guidelines and eat less fat, this trend could worsen. Yet this is what the pyramid suggests — eat fats sparingly. Even worse is the food pyramid recommendation promoting the use of margarine, which is made of hydrogenated and partially hydrogenated fat; its consumption can disrupt the balance of fats and promote more inflammation. For the endurance athlete, EFA imbalance can contribute to inflammatory conditions, poor recovery and chronic injury.

High-Glycemic Carbohydrates

The pyramid suggests that most foods consumed should be bread, cereal, rice and pasta — up to 11 servings a day! Most people consume carbohydrates in their processed form: white bread (including rolls, bagels and crackers), processed cereal (practically all the cereal on the market), white rice and white-flour pasta. These are among the most harmful foods in our society, contributing to heart disease, cancer, hypertension, diabetes and other diseases. These high-glycemic foods rapidly raise blood sugar and insulin, reduce our ability to burn fat, and add more stress to the adrenal glands.

Low Nutrient Levels

Assessments of the pyramid diet made by NutrAnalysis, Inc., show low and borderline levels of many vitamins and minerals. For example, a sample diet of a 52-year-old woman who consumed 1,600 calories based on the food pyramid had below-RDA levels of pantothenic acid, vitamins B6, B12 and E, biotin and the minerals chromium, copper, iodine, iron, magnesium, manganese, sodium and zinc. Borderline RDA levels included those in folic acid, calcium and potassium.

A 30-year-old female consuming 2,200 calories still had many below-normal levels of nutrients: pantothenic acid, vitamin B12, biotin, vitamin E, chromium, copper, manganese and zinc. Borderline levels included those from iodine, iron and magnesium. In a sample diet of a young male eating 2,800 calories, similar findings prevailed. Low or borderline levels included pantothenic acid, vitamin B12, biotin, vitamin E, chromium and copper.

The pyramid issue may best be summed up by Siguel: "The beneficiaries of this policy (the pyramid) are bureaucrats protecting their jobs, researchers studying low-fat foods, corporations selling low-fat foods to an uninformed and misled public, and companies selling drugs to lower abnormal cholesterol and hypertension caused by EFA deficiency. The losers are consumers faced with increasing health-care costs, abnormal cholesterol and chronic diseases including heart disease, as well as nutritionists and patients who face conflicting and misleading guidelines."

5

Fats, Oils and Endurance

Today's endurance athletes have been led to believe that carbohydrates are the key to endurance. Nothing could be further from the truth. As a matter of fact, carbohydrates can very easily restrict your energy for endurance. Fats — both the type stored in the body and fats and oils in the diet — are the real keys to greater endurance. And while dietary fats have been vilified as threats to overall health, much scientific and medical evidence indicates the contrary. This chapter discusses two important aspects of dietary fat:

- The quantity or total percentage of fat in the diet, and its effect on energy for endurance.
- The quality of fat and the proper ratio of different types of dietary fat, and their effects on overall health, including inflammation, injury, immunity and disease.

As discussed in previous chapters, fats can provide significant amounts of energy for endurance, and for many other daily functions of the body and its organs. For example, the heart may derive as much as 100 percent of its energy from fats. The importance of fat as a nutrient for energy in endurance athletes is well established in scientific and medical literature (see bibliography). The use of higher-fat diets (but not high-fat or excess-fat diets) to improve athletic performance in humans is also well supported in medical literature. These studies demonstrate that increasing dietary fat above the traditionally recommended levels, or levels typically consumed by athletes, significantly improved maximum oxygen uptake (VO_2 max), performance, endurance, carbohydrate sparing and resistance to fatigue. It should be noted that when dietary fat is increased, usually carbohydrate content is reduced.

Improved utilization of fats, which traditionally is said to take place at up to 60 percent of an individual's VO_2 max, was shown recently to take place at up to 80 percent VO_2 max when athletes consumed diets higher in fat. In these same athletes, 90 to 95 percent of their VO_2 max could be maintained, despite marked glycogen depletion. In addition to endurance, anaerobic power was also maintained in these athletes. These findings confirmed earlier studies in animals, as well as the observations I made during my initial work with athletes in the late 1970s.

In addition, high-fat diets can improve the response of growth hormone to exercise. Some athletes now attempt this by taking synthetic growth hormone, which is not only a banned substance in most sports, but is also unhealthy for the body.

The common recommendation is that dietary fat should be limited to 30 percent or less, as recommended by the National Cholesterol Education Program in 1991. However, many athletes attempt diets very low in fat, often in hopes of reducing body fat. This approach is quite often unsuccessful and will be discussed further in Chapter 18. Regarding this approach Gurndy states, in *Present Knowledge in Nutrition*, "one can question whether it is realistic, necessary, or strongly based on scientific data."

The World Health Organization suggests that dietary fat intake by athletes may be as high as 35 percent. Consuming a diet higher in fat, even in excess of 30 percent, can be accomplished without risk of cardiovascular or immune stress. In addition, studies have shown that women developed higher risk for heart disease with a lower-fat, higher-carbohydrate diet vs. a higher-fat, lower-carbohydrate diet. In addition to reducing triglyceride levels, higher-fat, lower-carbohydrate diets can improve insulin and blood-sugar balance.

Increasing the intake of dietary fat can increase an important enzyme called lipoprotein lipase, which makes fats more available for energy in muscles. However, consuming a diet too high in carbohydrates may diminish lipoprotein lipase and be associated with diminished ability to obtain energy from fats, and increased dependency on the very limited carbohydrate stores.

In general, female endurance athletes utilize more fats and less carbohydrates than men, and women store less glycogen from dietary carbohydrates than men. In this respect, women are relatively more efficient in endurance sports. Unfortunately, women are often the ones who strive to follow low-fat diets.

A variety of problems may be associated with low levels of fat intake. For example, amenorrheic female athletes consumed less fat (and more carbohydrate) than women athletes with normal menstrual cycles. The desire to be thin may influence dietary choices in these athletes. Low-fat diets have also been associated with significantly low testosterone levels in men. Various skin problems may also be related to low intake of dietary fat. Fat may also reduce pain; in one study, individuals in pain who ate high-fat (low-carbohydrate) meals reported significantly reduced pain 90 minutes after ingestion.

For many athletes, avoiding the low-fat approach can help increase energy for endurance. But just any fat is not sufficient. Eating the right types of fats, and in the proper balance, is also important.

Cholesterol

Whenever there's talk about increasing dietary fats, dietary and serum cholesterol is usually a concern. Cholesterol, like dietary fat, takes a bad rap in discussions about health, and is actually an important substance for proper functioning of all individuals, especially athletes. The production of key hormones depends upon cholesterol. This includes the glucocorticoids, which help regulate energy production, as well as estrogen, progesterone and testosterone. In addition, the production of bile, and the formation of vitamin D in the skin are dependent upon cholesterol. Cholesterol is also an important component of all cells, including those in the nervous system.

Most important to understand is that almost everyone has effective feedback-control mechanisms regarding cholesterol intake, with consumption of high levels of cholesterol not necessarily affecting blood levels. The body requires about 1,000 mg of cholesterol per day for normal function. Most of this is made by the liver, with only about 10 to 20 percent coming from the diet. If less cholesterol is consumed through foods, more is made by the liver, and if more is eaten, the liver produces less. Dysfunction in the liver may be the major reason for abnormal blood levels of cholesterol since it is here that cholesterol is broken down into bile salts and eliminated through the gall bladder and the intestine. In addition, low dietary-fiber intake may allow reabsorption of more cholesterol from the intestine after removal by the gall bladder.

Most concerns about cholesterol have to do with its relationship with cardiovascular heart disease (CHD). However, there are actually two types of cholesterol — HDL and LDL. Current evidence indicates that heart disease is related to a high LDL cholesterol fraction, while a high HDL fraction is related to a reduced risk of heart disease. It has also been shown that the oxidation of LDL cholesterol is a key factor in this process, and the use of antioxidants (discussed in Chapter 13) may play a role in preventing this problem. Some dietary fatty acids have been shown to raise LDL cholesterol:

- Palmitic, myristic and lauric acids, which are a significant part of foods high in saturated fat, raise LDL and total cholesterol. Foods high in these fatty acids include palm-kernel oil (78 percent), coconut oil (71 percent), herring (41 percent), palm oil (39 percent) and pork (30 percent),

- Stearic acid makes up about 25 percent of the saturated fat in the diet but does not raise LDL cholesterol. Higher levels of stearic acid are found in cocoa butter, pork and beef.

- Linoleic acid, an omega-6 fat, mildly lowers LDL cholesterol and is found in many oils.

- Trans fats (found in hydrogenated, overheated and rancid oils) increase LDL cholesterol and lower the beneficial HDL.

HDL cholesterol has positive effects on cardiac health, and low levels are associated with heart disease. High-carbohydrate diets may lower HDL cholesterol. In addition, fenugreek, an herb, can significantly decrease the total cholesterol and triglycerides without affecting the HDL. I have successfully used powdered fenugreek (Fen-Gre from Standard Process, Inc.) to lower high cholesterol, and, as a preventative measure, for those who have a family history of high cholesterol.

It is important when testing your blood that the total cholesterol, LDL and HDL fractions, are measured (along with triglycerides), in the fasting state. High triglyceride levels are also positively correlated with CHD. Omega-3 fats lower triglycerides, and carbohydrates raise triglycerides.

Balance of Fats

In addition to using fats for energy, the body also uses them for a variety of health benefits. Regarding this, it's important to consider that fat intake must be balanced. Broadhurst's statement in the journal *Medical Hypothesis* summarizes this issue well: "Natural whole foods contain fats as structural components, and have a balance of polyunsaturated fat, monounsaturated fat, and saturated fat. Since we are still a Paleolithic species, adapted to eating only wild foods, it is difficult to justify the consumption of anything other than an overall balance of (fats) in an evolutionary sense. No natural fats are intrinsically good or bad — it is the proportions that matter. Variety is recommended . . . (and) degree of saturation, and chain length. Pathological n-3/n-6 (omega-3/omega/6) polyunsaturated fat imbalance, obesity, and progressive glucose intolerance (carbohydrate intolerance) are consequences of adopting cereal-grain-based diets by both humans and livestock. Food processing and refining amplify these problems."

The Hormonal System

Our body produces many different hormones for health and fitness. But for this to take place, the process is dependent upon fat. Most important are the adrenal-gland hormones which help regulate electrolytes, water and the burning of fat and sugar for energy. In addition, the thymus gland regulates immunity and your body's defense systems; the thyroid regulates temperature, weight and other metabolic functions; the kidney's hormones help regulate blood pressure, circulation and filtering of blood. Without the right balance of fats in the system the hormonal system can't produce hormones.

Insulation

The body's ability to store the right amount of fat permits us to live in most climates, especially in areas of extreme heat and cold. In warmer areas of the world, stored fat provides protection from the heat; in colder regions, increased fat stored beneath the skin prevents too much heat from leaving the body.

An example of fat's effectiveness as an insulator is in the Eskimo's ability to withstand great cold and survive in good health. Eskimos eat a good deal of fat and much of it is stored under their skin. Moreover, despite a heavy diet of these fats, Eskimos have a very low incidence of heart and other disease.

A Natural Beauty Aid

Cholesterol also serves as an insulating barrier within the skin. Without this protection, water and water-soluble substances such as chemical pollutants would enter the body through the skin. It's the protective qualities of fat that give the skin the soft, smooth and unwrinkled appearance so many people try to achieve through expensive skin conditioners. The healthy look of skin comes from the fat inside. The same is true for your hair. With the proper balance and amounts of fats in your diet, your skin and hair develops a healthy appearance. In fact, if you've been looking for the ideal skin and hair product, you can end your search by balancing the fats in your diet.

Fat also prevents too much water from leaving the body, which can result in dehydration that causes dry, scaly skin. Some evaporation is normal, of course, but fats under the skin regulate the evaporation and can prevent as much as 10 to 20 times more water from leaving the body.

Pregnancy and Lactation

For many years doctors told women not to gain too much weight during pregnancy; 20 to 25 pounds was the maximum weight gain advised. Many women followed this advice by eliminating fats from their diets, which sometimes created nutritional deficiencies and problems with fat metabolism. This was unhealthy for both mother and baby.

Today, more doctors are recommending higher average weight gains during pregnancy. Depending on the woman's frame, and her health, up to 30 or more pounds is acceptable. This has been shown to result in healthier babies and mothers, so long as the mother is active in the months after birth.

The time to improve your health is long before you decide to have a baby. Being in a state of good health will also make conceiving a child much easier. This applies to males as well as females. The effective functioning of the hormonal system is important to both would-be parents. Once conception does take place, fats are important to the continued good health of the mother and child.

The uterus must maintain the health of the newly conceived embryo by providing nutrition until the placenta can begin to function, usually a period of a week or more. If there is an adequate level of progesterone, which is produced from fats, then there should be enough nutrients for the newly formed embryo to survive the first critical week. Without enough progesterone, the embryo could die.

And, the placenta must form and be in good functioning order, producing hormones that affect the developing fetus. Both of these hormones — estrogen and progesterone — are fat dependent and are produced in increasing quantities as the pregnancy continues. Together they promote the growth of the uterus and the storage of nutrients for the fetus. The proper development of the fetus has obvious hormonal relationships, which are dependent upon fats.

Following birth, breast feeding helps protects the baby against allergies, asthma and intestinal problems, through its high-quality fat content, especially cholesterol. Especially during the first few days, the baby is highly dependent on milk's fat for survival. During this first stage of breast-milk production, the high colostrum content is of vital nutritional importance. The uniqueness of breast milk has never been duplicated in any artificial formula.

X-Ray Protection

Fats seem to help protect the body against the harmful effects of X-rays. This occurs through physical protection of the cell, and by controlling production of free radicals, generated as a result of X-ray exposure. In addition to medical X-rays, we are exposed to X-rays from the atmosphere all the time. This cosmic radiation penetrates most objects, including airplanes. The average person gets more cosmic-radiation exposure during a airline flight from New York to Los Angeles than from an entire lifetime of medical X-rays.

Digestion

Because so many people digest their food poorly — a common result of stress — they do not always efficiently absorb the nutrients in foods. Lipase and bile are both fatty substances which aid in the digestion and absorption of fats and fat-soluble vitamins. If there is not enough fat in the diet, not enough bile will be secreted. It is the secretion of bile into the small intestine that makes fat in the diet digestible. Certain lipase-containing foods like avocados and green extra-virgin olive oil can greatly aid digestion of fats.

Fat in the meal also helps regulate the rate of stomach emptying, allowing for better digestion of proteins. If you are always hungry it may be because your meal is too low in fat and your stomach is emptying too rapidly. Fats also slow the absorption of sugar from the small intestines, which keeps insulin from rising too high and too quickly.

Support and Protection

Fats offer physical support and protection to vital body parts, acting like a natural, built-in shock absorber, cushioning our organs and glands from the wear and tear of everyday life, and preventing organs from sinking due to the downward pull of gravity. Fats also protect the inner lining of the stomach and intestines from irritating substances in the diet, such as alcohol and spicy foods. When the body-fat content is too low, these functions can have a negative impact on your overall health.

Vitamin and Mineral Regulation

Cholesterol's presence in the skin is involved with the reaction which results in the production of vitamin D. Sunlight chemically changes cholesterol through the process of irradiation to vitamin D. This newly formed vitamin D is necessary for the absorption of calcium and phosphorous. Without the vitamin D, calcium and phosphorous would not be well absorbed and deficiencies of both could occur. But without cholesterol, the whole process would not occur.

Once calcium is absorbed into the body it still needs to be taken into the bone or muscle cells. And that's where fat plays an essential role. In order for calcium to enter the bone or muscle, prostaglandins, made from fat, are needed; if there is not enough fat, then too little calcium may enter the bone and muscle. When that happens, the results can be stress fractures, osteoporosis, and collapsed vertebrae. When there's calcium in the blood but not enough entering the muscle cells because of a lack of a fat carrier, the muscles may get sore and stiff since calcium is needed to relax muscles. If the calcium is not used, it may contribute to calcium stores, sometimes in the kidneys as stones or in the muscles or joint spaces as calcium deposits. Other vitamins, including A, D, E and K, rely on fat for proper absorption and utilization. These important vitamins are fat dependent for three reasons:

- They are present in fatty foods in higher amounts. The body cannot make an adequate amount of these vitamins to ensure continued good health.

- These vitamins require fat in the intestines in order to be absorbed. A low-fat diet could be deficient in these vitamins to begin with and could restrict their absorption.

- Once absorbed, these vitamins require another substance to carry them through the blood, the lipoproteins, a combination of fat and protein. Again, fat is essential to the diet or these vitamins wouldn't get very far and wouldn't enhance our health.

Taste

My favorite function of fats is that they make food delightfully palatable. Let's face it, people love foods with fat in them, but are so guilt-ridden about it, they just can't sit down at the dinner table and enjoy them. Fats do not have to be an unhealthy addition to your diet if properly balanced. They not only taste good, but they make you feel good. And not just psychologically, but physiologically as well.

Fats also satisfy our physical hunger. People on low-fat diets often complain that they are always hungry. Well, of course they are — without fats in the diet, they can't achieve a feeling of satiety. As a result, the brain just keeps sending the same message over and over: eat more, eat more. Because you never really feel satisfied, the temptation to overeat is irresistible. In fact, there's a good chance you can actually gain weight on a low-fat diet by overeating to try and get that "I'm not hungry anymore" feeling. Besides, low-fat meals can be extremely unappetizing, often leading to an unbalanced diet. This problem is rampant in our geriatric population.

In addition to the use of fats for energy, and the important items just listed, fats are involved in the process of inflammation and the production of natural anti-inflammatory chemicals by your body. This is discussed in the next chapter.

6

Controlling Inflammation

The body produces inflammatory chemicals as a result of many activities — from typing and walking, to working out and racing. Any repetitive motion results in inflammation. This process is part of the recovery/healing mechanism, which also includes manufacturing natural anti-inflammatory hormones to counter those which are inflammatory. The natural fats in our diet play a vital role in this process. By balancing these fats, our inflammatory/anti-inflammatory mechanism also remains balanced.

The easiest way to understand the balance of fats is to use the ABC model: There are A fats, B fats and C fats which make up our diet. Each one goes through changes in your body, resulting in a series of chemicals called eicosanoids (made up of prostaglandins, leukotrienes and thromboxanes); A, B and C fats convert to series 1, 2 and 3 eicosanoids respectively.

A fats are found in most vegetables, and in the oils of safflower, peanut and corn. They are the more delicate fats, generally grown in warmer climates, and are sometimes referred to by their chemical name, omega-6. Most contain the essential fatty acid, linoleic acid (LA). It's essential because the body is not able to make it. You must get it from your diet — and without it you cannot be healthy. When consumed, LA is converted by the body to gamma-linolenic acid (GLA) and finally to the first series of prostaglandins we'll call PG1, along with other natural chemicals which collectively are called eicosanoids. Food concentrates of black currant seed oil, for example, are also in this category, are unique because they already contain the converted GLA, a key nutrient in fat metabolism. Black currant seed oil is useful as a nutritional supplement for individuals who require more omega-6 fats.

The B fats are the saturated ones, and contain the important fat arachondonic acid (AA). This fat is quickly converted to a prostaglandin we'll call PG2, and other natural eicosanoids. B fats have, in recent years, been mistaken for "bad" fats. They are found in dairy products, butter, meats and egg yolks. However, scientific evidence has not really implicated these as destructive to health when consumed as part of a balanced diet, despite what the TV commercials say. The famous Framingham study, for example, found no relationship between egg consumption, blood cholesterol and coronary heart disease (CHD). Yet people still avoid eating eggs. Undoubtedly, modern social trends and the marketing of fake foods such as margarine and imitation eggs are partly responsible. Cereal commercials tell us how healthy their products are despite being filled with sugar.

The C fats are found in fish and beans, and the oils from flaxseed and walnut. Chemically termed omega-3, this group also includes the food concentrates from flaxseed and fish oil (which contains eicosapentaenoic acid, or EPA). C fats are the hearty ones, originally produced in the northern climates. They contain the essential fatty acid alpha linolenic acid (ALA), which is converted in the body to EPA and finally to the third prostaglandin group, PG3 and other eicosanoids.

The most important aspect of this is that the series 2 eicosanoids produce our inflammatory chemicals, and the series 1 and 3 eicosanoids produce anti-inflammatory ones. Too much inflammation is, of course, a problem — it prevents recovery from workouts and races, maintains chronic injuries and ultimately could lead to disease. So it's important to eat a balance of A, B and C fats so as to make a balance of inflammatory and anti-inflammatory chemicals.

We should consume approximately equal amounts of each in the course of a day, week or month (not necessarily at each meal). If you are a vegetarian and do not consume many B fats, then you need to take in approximately an equal ratio of A and C fats; in this case, some of the A fats will be

UNDERSTANDING THE ABCs		
A fats	Series 1 eicosanoids	Anti-inflammatory and other effects
B fats	Series 2 eicosanoids	Inflammatory and other effects
C fats	Series 3 eicosanoids	Anti-inflammatory and other effects

converted to B fats, as discussed below. By eating a balance of all three fats, you also have an ideal ratio of unsaturated to saturated fats: 2:1.

By eating a balance of A, B and C fats, you're on your way to balancing the series 1, 2 and 3 eicosanoids, and properly regulating your body chemistry to avoid excess inflammation and injury. However, many athletes have imbalances in this mechanism — it was probably the most common problem I saw in athletes during my years in practice.

Imbalances can occur for several reasons main reasons:

- Eating too much of one type and/or not enough of another fat.
- A lack of certain nutrients — specific vitamins and minerals — which are required for the conversion of A and C fats to their respective eicosanoids
- Presence of certain dietary factors can inhibit the conversion of A and C fats to eicosanoids; other factors can have a positive effect.
- Lifestyle factors, such as stress, which prevent formation of series 1 and 3 eicosanoids. Even aging has an effect on this process.

Dietary Balance

The proper balance of fats was described above, but it's so important that I will mention it again here. If you do not properly balance your A, B and C fats, you'll have too much inflammation throughout the body, especially in areas you're most vulnerable. These ultimately become the sites of injury.

For example, if you eat too much meat and not enough vegetables, beans or fish, you may end up producing too many series 2 eicosanoids and too many inflammatory chemicals. Those with chronic inflammatory problems are often in this situation. Conditions with medical labels that end with the suffix "-itis" refer to inflammation.

Nutritional Needs

A variety of nutrients are necessary for the conversion of A and C fats to their respective eicosanoids. If these nutrients are not present, the series 1 and 3 eicosanoids will be reduced, leaving a relatively high level of series 2 eicosanoids — this means too much inflammation. For this reason, many inflammatory conditions respond well to supplementation with certain nutrients. The vitamins most important in this process include B6, niacin, and vitamin C. Vitamin E is also important but in low doses (see Chapter 12). In addition, specific minerals are also necessary. They include magnesium, zinc and calcium.

If you have inflammatory conditions, the first step in correcting the problem is to evaluate your diet to make sure you're getting the proper amount of these nutrients. If that's not the case, supplementation with the proper nutrients, in the proper form and dose, is essential (see Chapter 12).

Dietary Factors

There are two aspects of diet when considering inflammation; there are some items in our food supply which can promote inflammation, and others which can reduce it.

The most common food item which promotes an increase of series 2 and reduces series 1 and 3 eicosanoids are trans fats. This is an artificially manufactured fat found in hydrogenated and partially hydrogenated oils, as well as many oils which have been overheated such as in fried foods. The only good thing about this harmful substance is that its presence is usually listed on food labels. It's sometimes not listed when ingredients such as peanut butter are used. For example, many foods contain peanut butter which has added hydrogenated fat and even sugar. But those ingredients are not listed. Read labels carefully.

Margarine contains a lot of of trans fats, as do many packaged and prepared food items. These fats also behave as B fats, so not only do trans fats inhibit series 1 and 3 production, these fats increase the amount of B fats in your diet. While a trans fat begins as an A or C fat — soy oil, for example — it is processed in such a way as to change its molecular structure and now is a B fat. In addition, too much of any B fat in the diet can also promote inflammation.

In addition, other foods can disturb the delicate balance of fats promoting inflammation. Too much sugar (glucose and fructose), too much alcohol and low-protein diets can cause the same problems that too much B fat and trans fats produce: decreased series 1 and 3 eicosanoids with an increase in series 2.

The main reason why so many factors can affect the production of eicosanoids is due to the presence of a specific enzyme (called delta-6 desaturase). This important enzyme depends on the nutrients listed above for normal function, and are also protein-dependent. These enzymes are also inhibited — not allowed to function — in the presence of other related factors listed above.

The Aspirin Connection

Aspirin (acetylsalicylic acid), and other non-steroidal anti-inflammatory drugs (NSAIDs), are among the most commonly recommended and prescribed drugs in the world. Their use by athletes is especially common. However, their anti-inflammatory and analgesic (pain-reducing) effects are not without side effects. The most noteworthy is the potential for delayed tissue healing and other problems described below.

NSAIDs do their job by inhibiting another enzyme (cyclo-oxygenase) involved in eicosanoid production, and result in the reduction of not only the series 2 eicosanoids, but the series 1 and 3 as well. (This does not reduce all inflammation, but most.) In other words, if taking aspirin improves your inflammatory condition, it's through the action by aspirin of artificially, and temporarily, balancing the series 1, 2 and 3 eicosanoids. So when and if this happens, it means your eicosanoids were not balanced. In this situation, rather than rely on NSAIDs, aim to balance your eicosanoids by balancing your A, B and C fats and making sure all the factors are present that are important, and reduce those that interfere with the balance you are seeking.

As mentioned, NSAIDs are not without some very serious side effects. Among them is the slowing of the healing process. This is due to slowing of white blood cells coming to sites of injury, and other chemical effects including those in the immune system. This can not only delay tissue healing but also can impair scar formation, resulting in diminished strength of the mature scar. More importantly, NSAIDs may also inhibit the repair process in healing fractures, since the first critical stage of this process involves inflammation.

Another common side effect occurs in the intestine. NSAIDs are commonly associated with an increased incidence of gastric and duodenal ulcers, and always cause gastrointestinal bleeding. In addition, blood flow to the intestine can be reduced in those taking NSAIDs, which could affect digestion and especially absorption of nutrients.

There are also other adverse side effects of NSAIDs:

- The use of NSAIDs can produce muscle dysfunction, and exaggerated exercise-associated muscle damage.

- The consensus of studies does not show that NSAIDs adequately reduce delayed-onset muscle soreness (DOMS) — a common reason athletes use them.
- NSAIDs can adversely affect repair of joint cartilage. These effects are greater on arthritic cartilage than normal cartilage.
- NSAIDs can cause liver and kidney damage, especially in those who are dehydrated (a frequent problem in athletes, especially during long endurance workouts and races).
- Other side effects can include headaches, skin rash, tinnitus (ringing in the ears) and drowsiness.
- NSAIDs, especially aspirin, and ibuprofen, can interfere with normal sleep patterns, including suppression of melatonin and changes in body temperature.
- Reye's syndrome (a potentially fatal condition in children causing liver, neurological and mitochondrial damage) has been associated with aspirin and other salicylate use in conjunction with viral infections.

Oddly enough, many patients who take NSAIDs for pain and inflammation may not really need them. Dieppe and colleagues (1993) reported their study in the *British Journal of Rheumatology* demonstrating that 20 of 44 patients studied with osteoarthritis were able to stop their regular NSAID use without return of pain (and without other therapy).

It should be noted that acetaminophen (sold as Tylenol and Anacin 3) also has analgesic effects but does not have anti-inflammatory actions. Prolonged overuse or use with alcohol may result in liver damage.

Other Functions of Eicosanoids

In addition to controlling inflammation, the eicosanoids have many other important functions. The series 1 and 3 hormones decrease blood clotting and dilate blood vessels which lowers blood pressure and increases circulation. The series 2 eicosanoids, however, do almost the opposite; they constrict blood vessels thereby increasing blood pressure. They increase blood clotting, and can, when out of balance, trigger tumor growth, asthma and menstrual cramps. Even though we think of these as the "bad" eicosanoids because they are related to saturated fats, the fact is we need their actions. For example, without the constricting of blood vessels and the raising of blood pressure, our circulation would be poor and we would not get enough oxygen and other nutrients circulated to our cells, significantly reducing our energy for endurance. Or, without blood clotting, a small cut could cause us to bleed to death. So don't think of "good" and "bad." Think of balance.

Here are some other indications that there may be an imbalance in fats and the respective eicosanoids:

- If taking aspirin reduces your inflammation.
- In the spring, the body's normal levels or series 1 eicosanoids diminish. If low levels already exist, this time of year will be accompanied by symptoms, most commonly those associated with spring allergies.
- Large-intestine function is also related to fat balance; too much series 2 eicosanoids may increase constipation, too much series 1 may produce diarrhea.
- Ulceration of the GI track is also associated with low levels of series 1 or 3 eicosanoids. These normally serve a protective function in the lining of the intestine.
- My experience with individuals who are overfat and/or overweight indicates there is often a need for series 3 eicosanoids.

The delta-5 Enzyme

In addition to the enzymes which convert A and C fats to their respective eicosanoids, another enzyme can potentially cause problems when in excess. The delta-5 desaturase enzyme can cause A fats to be converted to B fats. This can be disastrous, and is the reason why some authorities note that both A and B fats can be harmful if in excess.

Excessive amounts of this enzyme may be due to the hormone insulin, which itself can be produced in excess with high carbohydrate intakes. Thus, high-carbohydrate foods increase insulin, which converts more A fats to B fats, which in turn makes more series 2 eicosanoids which are inflammatory.

Both EPA (from fish oil) and sesamin (a substance in raw, unheated sesame oil) can prevent this from happening by inhibiting the delta-5 enzyme. This is another way you can balance your eicosanoids, by eating enough fish and raw sesame seeds. Unfortunately, most people don't do this. Moreover, much of the high-EPA fish (like salmon) comes from fish farms, which do not contain much EPA (in natural waters, fish feed on plankton which is how they make EPA. The water in fish farms does not contain plankton). And, most sesame seeds consumed are toasted, or otherwise heated.

Fish-oil supplements (EPA) and unrefined sesame seed oil capsules are most useful to help balance eicosanoids. These are especially useful for athletes who are increasing their training volume or intensity, and especially during competition since these are the activities which result in more inflammation. These are discussed further in Chapter 11.

7

Carbohydrates and Endurance

Today athletes are bombarded with advertisements that promise more energy through sugar-laden foods, drinks and gels. While companies know just how far to go before landing on the Federal Trade Commission's carpet for false advertising, they make their point that energy comes from sugar. And in the advertisement game, whoever has the most money wins. So large companies spend billions of dollars to persuade you to eat more sugar in hopes of getting that energy. Unfortunately, what you're not told is the energy that comes from sugar is very short-lived, and not appropriate when it comes to energy for endurance, except *during* long activity.

Concentrated carbohydrates include foods such as bread and other items made from any type of flour, including rolls, muffins, pancakes and pasta, as well as cereal, rice, potatoes, fruit and fruit juice, soft drinks, and of course, sugar itself and foods containing sugar in all forms. Most foods contain some carbohydrates. Some foods don't seem to contain much sugar, but a closer look reveals otherwise. For example, many popular fruit yogurts contain 7 teaspoons of sugar per serving — these yogurts are loaded with more sugar per serving than most ice cream! Foods like ketchup, and many prepared or packaged foods, also contain lots of sugar.

Reading the labels may help you find the sugar listed in the ingredients. However, you must realize that sugar is often disguised in foods under its many aliases, including sucrose, fructose, dextrose, lactose, maltose, barely malt and glucose. In addition, corn syrup, high-fructose corn syrup and maltodextrin (these are all just corn syrup) are just other fancy names for sugar.

Even some artificial sweeteners actually contain sugar. Worse yet, some companies even promote sugars such as maltodextrin as if they have some special qualities. They don't. It's all sugar.

Consuming large amounts of sugar (it all adds up) or, for many athletes, even moderate amounts of sugar can impair energy for endurance. Unfortunately, most athletes probably already consume too much sugar. If you follow the current USDA recommendations, you're eating two cups of sugar each day! And that's not counting those sweets you sneak in.

Insulin's Effect

Much of the utilization of dietary carbohydrate centers on the production of insulin. Following absorption of glucose (from dietary carbohydrates) into the blood, insulin has three major effects on this blood glucose (or blood sugar):

- Approximately 50 percent is utilized for energy in our cells.
- 40 percent or more is converted to fat.
- Up to 10 percent is stored as glycogen.

Insulin can cut into your health and endurance like a double-edged sword — converting dietary carbohydrates into fat stores while simultaneously inhibiting the utilization of stored fat for energy. Most importantly, a low-fat, high-carbohydrate diet can cause excess insulin production in relatively healthy athletes. In many unhealthy individuals, excess insulin is also a problem and may result even from moderate carbohydrate intakes.

It's also worth mentioning that excess insulin (called hyperinsulinemia) and high-carbohydrate diets have also been implicated as factors leading to many diseases, including heart disease, stroke, high blood pressure, breast cancer and diabetes.

How Much is Too Much

Other than to obtain fiber, it is generally believed by many scientists that humans have no true requirement for concentrated carbohydrates, since fat and protein can be converted to glucose. However, most athletes consume carbohydrates as their predominant macronutrient — typically 60 to 70 percent or more of their total intake. This is a problem not only because it means the intake of essential fats (the omega-6 and omega-3 previously mentioned) is restricted or sometimes eliminated, but also because protein intake is also reduced, sometimes significantly (the importance of protein is discussed in the next chapter). In addition, too much carbohydrate can produce too much insulin, which, as noted above, can impair your energy for endurance, diminish the body's fat-burning potential and cause your body to store more fat.

The Glycemic Index

The quality of a carbohydrate food is also an important factor to consider, and is referred to as the glycemic index (GI). The GI is a general measure of a carbohydrate food's ability to raise blood sugar, and the associated production of insulin. When a food with a high glycemic index is eaten, blood sugar rises more quickly, and insulin is produced in greater quantity. In general, processed carbohydrate foods have a higher glycemic index, and whole, unprocessed ones have a lower glycemic index (although this is not always true). In addition, other foods in your meal can lower the glycemic index of that meal, including its fat, protein and fiber content.

Lower-glycemic foods produce greater satiety — more of a feeling of fullness without the immediate hunger — than high-glycemic foods. A number of different studies have resulted in an extensive list of foods and their glycemic index. Appendix A lists foods from one of the more comprehensive lists. Note that juices usually have a much higher GI compared to the whole fruit. For example, whole grapefruit has a GI of 36, while grapefruit juice rates a 69.

High-quality, low-glycemic carbohydrates such as whole-grain foods, and whole fruits, rather than lower-quality high-glycemic foods such as sweets and white-flour products such as bagels, rolls, muffins, and fruit juice may also affect athletic performance. Studies show that low-glycemic foods resulted in higher concentrations of energy substrates, even after the exercise, including more-stable blood-sugar levels. The bottom line: real food, minimally processed, will give you more energy for endurance.

It has been known for many years that carbohydrate consumption before exercise may have a detrimental effect on endurance. However, the concept that muscle-glycogen depletion as the cause of exercise fatigue — a notion popular in the '60s, '70s and '80s — is only now being challenged in the '90s. In addition, it is now known that carbohydrate "loading" prior to exercise does not necessarily result in sparing muscle glycogen stores as once thought. Moreover, excess consumption of carbohydrate has been demonstrated to inhibit the use of fats for energy, which do spare glycogen. Studies have shown glucose and maltodextrin consumed before workouts forces your body to burn more sugar and less fat.

Another common routine among endurance athletes is consuming large amounts of carbohydrates immediately following exercise or competition in an attempt to replenish depleted glycogen stores. However, recent studies found that a mixed meal of carbohydrate, protein and fat will accomplish the same.

Carbohydrate Intolerance

The inability to properly metabolize the amount of carbohydrate in your diet is referred to as carbohydrate intolerance (CI). The problem occurs because of an excess production of the hormone insulin, which converts much of this carbohydrate food to body fat, and has other health consequences.

Here is a list of 10 most common complaints by people with CI and its advanced condition, insulin resistance. Many symptoms occur immediately following a meal containing too many carbohydrates, and others are constant.

- **Physical fatigue.** Whether you call it fatigue or exhaustion, the most common feature of CI is that it wears people out. Some are tired just in the morning or afternoon; others are exhausted all day. This tiredness may be different from the fatigue of adrenal stress and aerobic deficiency, but most often all of these problems occur together.
- **Mental fatigue.** Sometimes the fatigue is mental; the inability to concentrate is the most evident symptom. Loss of creativity, poor memory, and failing or poor grades in school often accompany CI, as do various forms of "learning disabilities." This fatigue is much more pronounced immediately after a meal. The worker who returns to his or her job site after lunch, only to be unable to concentrate due to mental fatigue, is common.
- **Low blood sugar.** Brief periods of low blood sugar are normal during the day, especially if meals are not eaten on a regular schedule. But prolonged periods of severe hypoglycemia, accom-

panied by many of the symptoms listed here, are not normal. Feeling jittery, agitated and moody is common in people with CI, with an almost immediate relief once food is eaten. Dizziness is also common, as is the craving for sweets, chocolate or caffeine. These bouts occur more frequently between meals. The old hypoglycemic diet, still in use today, recommends frequent snacks, and some individuals with CI usually know to eat often. However, the traditional hypoglycemic diet contains too much carbohydrate for most CI people.

- **Intestinal bloating.** Most intestinal gas is produced from dietary carbohydrates. CI sufferers who eat too much carbohydrates have lots of gas. Antacids are not very successful in dealing with the problem. The gas tends to build and is worse later in the day and at night.

- **Sleepiness.** Many people with CI get sleepy immediately after meals containing more than their limit of carbohydrates. This is typically a pasta meal, or even a meat meal which includes bread or potatoes, and a dessert.

- **Increased fat storage and weight**. Many people have too much stored body fat. In males, an increase in abdominal fat — the "carbo belly" — is the earliest sign of CI. In females, it's more prominent in the upper body compared to the thighs and legs. In the face, "chipmunk cheeks" is a telltale sign.

- **Increased triglycerides.** High triglycerides in the blood are often seen in overweight persons. But even those who are not yet fat may have stores of fat in their arteries as a result of CI. These triglycerides are the direct result of dietary carbohydrates being converted by insulin into fats called triglycerides. In my experience, fasting triglyceride levels of more than 100 may be an indication of a carbohydrate problem, (even though 100 is still in the so-called normal range). Triglyceride levels of more than 150 are diagnostic for insulin resistance.

- **Increased blood pressure.** Most people with hypertension produce too much insulin and are CI. As insulin levels elevate, so does blood pressure. For some people with CI, sodium sensitivity is common; eating too much sodium then causes water retention and may also raise blood pressure.

- **Depression.** Because carbohydrates are a natural "downer," potentially depressing the brain, it is not uncommon to see many depressed persons who are CI. Carbohydrates do this by increasing serotonin, a neurotransmitter made in the brain. Too much serotonin may produce a depressing or sleepy feeling. This is why some hotels put candy on your pillow in the evening; it literally helps you sleep.
- **Addictions.** CI is also prevalent in persons addicted to alcohol, caffeine, cigarettes or other drugs. Often, the drug is the secondary problem, with CI being the primary one. Treating this primary problem should obviously be a major focus of any therapy.

People most vulnerable to CI include those under stress, including overtraining, those taking estrogen and those with a family history of diabetes, heart disease and stroke. In addition, increasing age is frequently accompanied by an increase in CI.

If CI becomes chronic and insulin resistance increases, this functional problem can lead to heart disease, stroke, high blood cholesterol and diabetes, to name a few.

If you are carbohydrate intolerant, one of the most important things for you to know is your limits of carbohydrate intake. In Chapter 14 we'll discuss the Two-Week Test, which will help you find and set your limits for carbohydrate consumption.

8

Protein Power

Like carbohydrates and fats, protein requirements are relative to each individual athlete. While protein contributes only a small amount of energy — up to 15 percent of your exercise needs — it serves other important roles in helping to enhance endurance.

How much protein do you need? Here's the simple answer; once you determine your carbohydrate limits, and add in about 30 percent balanced fats, the rest of your diet is protein. As simple as this seems, this is usually the best amount of protein.

Protein is a major component of cell structure, including the muscles, and vital for enzymes, such as those necessary for the production of anti-inflammatory hormones described in Chapter 5. Many amino acids can be converted to glucose when either blood glucose or glycogen levels are low.

Daily protein requirements for adults are established by the World Health Organization (WHO) at 0.75g per kg body weight for Western diets. Some individual countries have modified this recommendation; the U.S. to 0.8g, Canada to 0.86g, Germany and Australia to 1.0g. Without performing a dietary analysis, however, these numbers may be much less useful.

How much protein is this amount, in terms of foods? The chart below lists approximately how much protein-rich food you'd have to eat for the desired protein intake for a 150-pound athlete:

It is important to understand that other foods not rich in protein also contribute to your daily protein needs. For example, a half cup of soy beans contains more than 30 grams of protein, a half cup of kidney beans about 7

PROTEIN INTAKE	AMOUNT OF PROTEIN	APPROXIMATE AMOUNT OF PROTEIN FOODS
0.8g/kg	**56 grams**	2 eggs (12), 1 serving roast beef (30), 3 oz. cheese (14).
1.0g/kg	**70**	2 eggs (12), 1 serving roast beef (30), 1.5 oz. cheese (7), shrimp cocktail (21).
1.2g/kg	**84**	2 eggs (12), 3 slices bacon (6), 1 serving roast beef (30), 3 oz. cheese (14), shrimp cocktail (21).
1.4g/kg	**98**	3 eggs (18), 2 slices Canadian bacon (12), 1 serving roast beef 30), 1/2 cup cottage cheese (17), shrimp cocktail (21).
1.6g/kg	**112**	2 eggs (12), 3 slices bacon (6), 1 serving roast beef (30), 1/2 cup cottage cheese (17), shrimp cocktail (21), 1 serving salmon (25).
1.8g/kg	**126**	3 eggs (18), 2 slices Canadian bacon (12), 1 serving roast beef (30), 1/2 cup cottage cheese (21), shrimp cocktail (21), 1 serving salmon (25).
2.0g/kg	**140**	3 eggs (18), 2 slices Canadian bacon (12), 1 serving roast beef (30), 1/2 cup cottage cheese (21), shrimp cocktail (21), 1 serving salmon (25), 3 slices turkey (15).

grams, and an ounce of mixed nuts 4 to 5 grams. And most vegetables contain a couple of grams, and if you're eating six servings a day that would add up to 12 grams. However, these protein foods are not complete proteins as discussed below.

Many experts are calling for major revisions to the standard protein recommendations. Specific proposals include much higher amounts for athletes because low intakes of protein may have a detrimental effect on performance. Lemon, in a 1996 *Nutrition Reviews* paper, states that "an increasing number of studies have appeared that indicate dietary protein needs are elevated in individuals who are regularly physically active. Together, these data suggest that the RDA for those who engage in regular endurance exercise should be about 1.2 to 1.4 grams of protein per kilogram of body mass per day (150-175 percent of the current RDA) and 1.7 to 1.8 grams of protein per kilogram of body mass per day (212-225 percent of the current RDA) for strength exercisers."

Lemon is not the only expert who has researched protein needs. Others have shown that:

- Daily protein intakes as high as 2 grams per kilogram may still be inadequate in athletes training at 64 percent of their VO_2 max.
- Endurance athletes may require protein intakes higher than bodybuilders. The increased use of amino acids and higher mitochondria in aerobic muscle fibers of endurance athletes increase their needs for protein.
- Greater gains in body mass occur during heavy resistance training in young men when 3.3 versus 1.3 grams of protein per kilogram per day are consumed.
- Negative nitrogen balance may occur in young men engaged in resistance training while consuming dietary protein at the RDA.
- The Canadian Recommended Nutrient Intake (RNI) for protein of 0.86 gram per kilogram per day is insufficient for athletes.
- Low protein intakes results in a loss of lean body mass and decreased power.
- Women eating too little protein experience significant losses in lean tissue, poor immune response and muscle dysfunction.
- Athletes at greatest risk for consuming insufficient protein include those on calorie-restricted diets, vegetarians and young athletes who are still growing.
- After a low-protein meal, amino acids in the blood and muscle decrease continuously for up to five to seven hours.

Why so many diverse opinions on protein requirements? In part, it's due to the word "requirement," which is used in different ways by different researchers. Fortunately, you can avoid all the confusion by finding your own individualized protein needs rather than following the same general recommendations for everyone.

There is much less evidence that daily protein intakes above 2 grams per kilogram of body weight is beneficial, with the potential of negative effects. Excess protein, including that used for energy, is converted to fat and stored. There may also be increased nutritional needs associated with high protein intakes; because vitamin B6, B12 and folic acid are involved in the metabolism of protein, increased protein intake may increase the requirements for these nutrients. Increased water intake may be required in those with higher protein intakes since excretion of higher nitrogen from the kidney may require more water. Excess protein may produce metabolic stress on liver and kidney function. The studies demonstrating these potential problems, however, have been done on patients with previously impaired kidney function. Long-term feeding of healthy animals with very high protein intakes has been shown in one study to have no adverse effects. The concerns regarding high protein intake and calcium loss may only occur with purified protein, and those associated with atherosclerosis, and may not apply to most humans.

As discussed in the next chapter, the essential amino-acid content of food is important. Foods containing the highest-quality protein contain a balance of essential amino acids. In this regard, the ideal protein food is egg, which is also among the highest level of digestibility, with whey and beef also being among the highest-quality proteins. However, lower-quality protein foods can be properly balanced, or combined, to provide the same nourishment as high-quality proteins. For example, a combination of cereal and a legumes provides a high-quality protein meal. It is not necessary to create a high-quality protein combination at each meal, but rather in the course of the day or week. However, with these combinations of food may come higher carbohydrate intakes.

Protein requirements may be influenced by digestion, absorption and caloric intake. The first step in protein utilization is efficient digestion to its individual amino acids, which can then be followed by absorption. Kilocalorie intake has a significant influence on protein needs; low kilocalorie diets may increase protein needs, and adequate kilocalories may reduce protein needs.

An important relationship exists between dietary protein and reactions by the immune system. Absorption of intact proteins may produce allergic or hypersensitivity reactions in some patients. This response results in the production of IgG, IgA and IgE antibodies, and can be measured in the serum of these individuals. Common allergens include proteins from cow's milk, wheat gluten and corn.

Complete vs. Incomplete Protein

As previously described, proteins are made up of amino acids. Traditionally, amino acids are grouped as either "essential" (not made by the body and must be consumed in the diet) or "non-essential" (can be manufactured within the body). However, all the amino acids are necessary for normal body function — even those referred to as "non-essential." All the amino acids are listed below:

Essential	Nonessential
Arginine[1]	Alanine
Histidine[1]	Asparagine
Isoleucine	Aspartate
Leucine	Cysteine
Lysine	Glutamate
Methionine	Glutamine[2]
Phenylalanine	Glycine
Threonine	Proline
Tryptophan	Serine
Valine	Tyrosine

[1]May be considered "semi-essential" as it is synthesized at rates inadequate to support growth in children.

[2]May be considered "conditionally essential" under conditions of stress.

The normal terminology with amino acids incorporates a "D" or an "L" before the name. For example, you may see glutamine listed as "L-glutamine." Only "L" amino acids occur in protein. Some "D" amino acids occur in nature, such as in antibiotics, and may also be manufactured by microorganisms. In this book, the amino acids referred to are those found in proteins and the "L" terminology will be understood.

The essential/non-essential terminology can be very misleading for two important reasons:

- The production of so-called non-essential amino acids requires other nutritional substances.
- Lower levels of these other nutritional substances could result in lower levels of non-essential amino acids.

Maintaining normal levels of essential amino acids is accomplished by eating and absorbing them from your diet and does not require further biochemical conversions requiring other nutrients and enzymes when used for protein synthesis. However, these amino acids do require numerous vitamins and minerals for their conversions into other active compounds (i.e., chemicals for the brain and nervous-system communications).

Examples of non-essential amino acids and the nutrients required to make them include: glutamine, which requires magnesium; serine, which requires niacin; and glycine, which requires choline. In other cases, some non-essential amino acids require essential amino acids for their production: cysteine (non-essential) is produced from methionine (essential), and serine (non-essential), which requires niacin.

Considering the above, effective levels of non-essential amino acids may be more difficult to attain compared to essential amino acids when a typical Western diet is followed. This has led some experts to argue that the non-essential amino acids are more important for your body than the essential ones, since humans have evolved lacking the ability to make our own non-essential amino acids.

It should also be noted that under high training volumes or intensities, and during the racing season, the need for some non-essential amino acids may rise. For example, in these situations, glutamine requirements may be much higher than normal. As discussed below, glutamine levels are low in overtrained athletes.

Protein Ingredients

When the need to increase protein exists, be careful about which protein sources you eat. Many proteins used in packaged foods — bars, drinks, protein tablets and other supplements — are highly processed. Processing of protein may result in the production of monosodium glutamate (MSG, that salty flavor enhancer used in Chinese restaurants), which has a bad reputation. Many people are allergic to it, and may not realize it. The Food and Drug Administration (FDA) acknowledges the presence of MSG in these foods, but does not require it to be listed in the ingredients on the label because the MSG is not added by the manufacturer in the form of pure MSG. That leaves us to understand which ingredients contain this potentially harmful substance so we can avoid them. The following ingredients always contain MSG:

- All isolates (like soy isolates, protein isolates, milk isolates, and whey isolates)
- All caseinates (like calcium caseinate and sodium caseinate)
- Ingredients labeled as textured protein or hydrolyzed protein.
- Low-fat milk products may also include milk solids that contain MSG.

Reactions to MSG, which may occur immediately or any time within 48 hours, can vary greatly in individual people. The symptoms may include flu-like achiness, joint pain, stiffness, depression, anxiety, hyperactivity, intestinal discomfort, skin rash and many others.

9

Water, Water, Everywhere

The most common nutritional deficiency in athletes is not one of the three most-commonly discussed macronutrients — carbohydrates, fats and proteins — but rather a fourth and most essential macronutrient: water. Despite the fact that drinkable water is readily available, many athletes are deficient in this important ergogenic aid that makes up about 60 percent of their bodies. When this percentage is lowered even slightly by dehydration, the result is poorly functioning muscles, blood and organs. Even a deficiency of less than 1 percent can bring on signs and symptoms of dysfunction.

Water may be the only added ergogenic requirement during activities lasting up to about 60 to 90 minutes, depending upon the individual. In prolonged activities, sodium is important, especially in hot environments. And macronutrients — especially carbohydrates — may serve an added role in maintaining fat-burning during long endurance workouts or competitions. But these do not replace the need for water.

Many athletes do not drink enough water between and during workouts and races. This is especially true in those who perform very long workouts; in these athletes maintaining normal hydration is even more difficult.

A young male athlete's body is typically 60 percent water, and may contain 42 kilograms (more than 92 pounds) of water. A female athlete's body is slightly less aqueous at 50 percent of total weight. Approximately, two-thirds of this water is in the intracellular areas — predominantly the muscles, with most of the remaining one-third in extracellular compartments in the blood.

One problem we have is our inability to easily know when water intake is needed. Generally, athletes wait for their sense of thirst to signal that it's time to drink. However, thirst is sensed only after dehydration has started.

Thirst is activated only when the total body-water level is reduced, and also by sodium levels as discussed in the next chapter. Even slight dehydration reduces the blood-plasma volume, which is really what triggers thirst. But thirst is sensed after dehydration is evident. More importantly, once you are dehydrated, it may take as much as 48 hours to properly rehydrate. This is why so many athletes, unknowingly, are in a constant state of dehydration.

As blood volume becomes diminished, blood flow (along with oxygen and other nutrients) to the muscles is significantly reduced, rendering them less functional. This condition raises the heart rate. Many athletes who observe an elevation of resting heart rate, or a plateau or worsening in their aerobic function are dehydrated. Their elevated heart rate forces them to slow the pace.

In addition, the ability to expel heat, which is always accumulating during training (and especially racing) is diminished by dehydration since skin circulation is reduced. This elevates the body's core temperature, which further reduces performance. This situation can also be dangerous.

If you have a difficult time getting into the habit of drinking often, use the alarm or countdown timer on your chronograph watch. If you work on a computer you may be able to set its alarm to remind you to drink while working. Set the alarm to remind you to drink every 60 to 90 minutes when at rest. During longer training efforts or races, you may wish to set the alarm on your watch to remind you to drink every 15 to 30 minutes, depending on your individual needs.

Sources of Water

Approximately 60 percent of your body's need for water comes from liquids, and 30 percent from foods. The other 10 percent is produced in the body from the metabolism of carbohydrates, fats and proteins as described in Chapter 1. The greatest water loss at rest, 60 percent, occurs from the kidneys. The remainder is lost through respiration — with equal amounts from skin and lungs totaling 30 percent, sweating accounting for 5 percent and large intestine function using another 5 percent. During exercise, however, sweating increases significantly, accounting for 90 percent of water loss — 1 to 2 liters per hour in prolonged training or competition.

If the water loss becomes greater than the intake, blood volume diminishes with significant adverse effects mentioned above. An endurance runner, for example, can expect his pace to be reduced by 2 percent for each percent of body weight lost by dehydration. Water losses of 6 to 10 percent may exist in marathon events, and losses can be even greater in longer competitions. This translates to a runner performing a 10 km race in 35 minutes under normal hydration, slowing to complete the same distance in almost 38 minutes when 4 percent dehydrated — a significant loss of performance. An Ironman event may take three additional hours with this amount of dehydration!

In athletes with better aerobic function, water regulation is more efficient, including maintenance of body temperatures and lower sweat rates. This is another reason to focus on building a great aerobic system, beginning in the off season (see *Training for Endurance*).

Athletes must develop the habit of drinking water each and every day, throughout the day, no matter the time of year. Don't wait until an upcoming event. The best advice is to drink small amounts of water — 4 to 6 ounces — throughout the day, every day. In a typical athlete, I suggest between 3 and 4 liters per day as a minimum. For larger athletes, more water will be needed. This does not include what is taken during workouts. Also, in athletes who work out more than a couple of hours, additional water may be required.

It's important to note that drinking large amounts of water at one time can inhibit thirst and promote a diuretic response. This may result, over time, in a lower net water volume in your body.

During hot days of training or racing, drinking additional water — 400-600 ml (13-20 ounces) — within 30 minutes of starting, may significantly delay dehydration and rises in body temperature. Be sure to experiment with this during training to know how far from the start and how much water you can drink without risking gastrointestinal distress.

Cool fluids, between 15 degrees and 22 degrees Centigrade (59 degrees and 72 degrees Fahrenheit) empty from the stomach more quickly than body-temperature fluids. Some athletes think this means drinking very cold fluids, but this may stimulate stronger stomach contractions creating gastrointestinal discomfort. So avoid ice water.

Another important consideration is how to drink water. Sounds easy, you've done it since you were an infant. But many athletes drink water in such a way as to swallow large amounts of air along with the water. If this is a problem for you, practice swallowing water during your training sessions. If you have trouble swallowing water without taking in air, it's often due to the placement of your tongue during swallowing. When drinking, the tip of your tongue should push against the back of your upper front teeth, with the middle of your tongue hitting the roof of your mouth.

Studies have demonstrated that observing the color of your urine is a good general guide for hydration status. A definite yellow color can indicate dehydration. Clear urine characterizes proper hydration. This approach, however, does not preclude the use of more-precise laboratory evaluations.

Another way to self-analyze yourself is to record each time you urinate during the day. If you're not urinating seven or eight or more times in a day, you're probably not drinking enough water.

Athletes may wish to avoid fluoridated water as well as the fluoride in toothpaste because fluoride inhibits an enzyme called enolase, which is important in converting carbohydrates to energy. Chlorinated water is also not recommended because of potential harmful side effects.

Also note that some food items can cause water loss from the body. Caffeine is the biggest culprit — from coffee, tea, cola, or even chocolate if you eat a lot of it. Caffeine is discussed in the next chapter.

10

Electrolytes

Nearly as important as water are the electrolytes — sodium, chloride, potassium, and magnesium. Of these, the sodium, chloride and potassium are discussed here, with magnesium being addressed later in Chapter 12.

Sodium and its associate chloride are the dominant electrolytes in the fluids surrounding our cells, with potassium being dominant inside the cell. Electrolyte regulation is controlled by sodium, which also helps regulate water balance, its intake through the diet, certain hormones (especially those made by the adrenal glands), and the nervous system.

Dietary intake of sodium, and its loss from the body, helps regulate both the thirst and salt appetite mechanism in the brain, with influence of certain kidney hormones. To help maintain rehydration for some hours after water ingestion, as a precompetition solution for example, drinks or foods should contain moderate levels of sodium. For example, the liberal use of sodium in your breakfast can help with your hydration during your workout or race.

A specific adrenal hormone, aldosterone, is important for electrolyte regulation, helping the body to hold on to sodium, and remove potassium. Adrenal dysfunction may reduce the body's sodium-retention mechanism. This is a common problem in athletes who are overtrained or under stress. This can result in excess sodium loss, excess potassium, and dehydration.

Aldosterone also affects sweat-gland function; it causes the body to retain its sodium and chloride, and allows the loss of some potassium. Nonetheless, most electrolytes lost in sweat are sodium and chloride.

Adrenal dysfunction can reduce aldosterone. In addition, this adrenal hormone causes increased sodium absorption from the intestine. With reduced aldosterone, diarrhea may result, causing significant losses of sodium and water.

Common conditions such as "athlete's diarrhea" are often due to chronic adrenal dysfunction — a problem which may not be evident until the stress of competition. This is especially true in those competing in longer events. Diarrhea in athletes may also be related to excess stress in the nervous system, which often exists in later stages of overtraining. The loss of sodium during adrenal dysfunction has also long been considered the reason for salt cravings in some athletes. The balance of dietary fats also has an influence on sodium balance through activity of the eicosanoids.

Low sodium levels — called hyponatremia — can occur during or after competitive events and can sometimes even be observed in a normal blood test in athletes who show no symptoms of hyponatremia. This means hyponatremia could exist in a symptomatic or asymptomatic state. Early symptoms may include weakness or disorientation. In extreme cases, hyponatremia can result in such problems as rapid neurological deterioration, cardiovascular instability and seizures.

The use of sodium during competition can be important, especially in long endurance events, as hyponatremia can occur if too much water and too little sodium is consumed. Small amounts of sodium added to water speeds stomach emptying of water and its absorption from the intestine. The American College of Sports Medicine's position on sodium is to include it in your drinks during workouts lasting longer than one hour to help promote fluid retention, and possibly preventing hyponatremia in certain individuals who drink excessive quantities of fluid. Use sea salt, and sprinkle it into your water bottle until only a very slight taste of salt is noticed.

Sodium tablets can be used during endurance events. The well-hydrated athlete sucks on a salt tablet (available in drug stores) until he or she loses the desire or taste for salt. In some cases, athletes consume many salt tablets during events of very long duration. In one case an athlete consumed more than 25 tablets while completing an Ironman-distance triathlon in a personal best time and place, and for the first time did not develop muscle cramps.

While large amounts of salt have been given to healthy individuals with no adverse effects, a very few individuals may be sodium sensitive. If this is the case, you'll notice that even small amounts of sodium added to your food produce fluid retention (typically swelling in the ankles) and can also raise blood pressure.

Especially for endurance athletes, severe hyponatremia and dehydration are the only two common potentially life-threatening medical emergencies. Avoidance of these can be accomplished by maintaining a state of optimal health and fitness. This means seeking normal adrenal function, consuming a diet that best matches your needs, and consuming proper fluid and electrolyte intake during competition and long training workouts.

In addition to sodium and chloride, potassium supplementation may also be necessary for athletes, although this is much less common. As a general guide, however, when adrenal function (i.e., aldosterone) is diminished, there is more sodium lost and the potassium levels are then excessive. It's important to note that excess potassium may be involved with the amplification of pain.

Sports Drinks and Gels

There are many ready-made and powdered sports drinks on the market, with a variety of marketing tactics advertising their benefits. They include many types of glucose or glucose-polymer drinks, some with or without various combinations of electrolytes and other nutrients. Unfortunately, most contain little or no sodium. Only plain water matches the needs of every athlete. In most cases, sports drinks are useful only during or immediately following longer training or competition, and should not be used to supplement the normal diet, nor as a replacement for a meal. Short workouts of an hour or less require only water for most athletes, although those with very good aerobic function can train much longer with plain water because so much of their energy is derived from fat.

As previously discussed, consuming large amounts of carbohydrates in drinks before workouts or competitions can have an adverse effect on performance. However, during long endurance events, like a marathon, long triathlon or any ultramarathon event, most likely both carbohydrate and electrolyte intake will be required.

Gel products are also used by some athletes and are a modified version of a sports drink without the water. They are very concentrated, sometimes with other nutrients added. Like carbohydrate and electrolyte drinks, they are not replacements for water. Because they are not made up predominantly of water, a user may require more water intake when using gels, especially during long workouts or competitions.

Other recommendations for fluids during and following activity can vary with each athlete. Some endurance athletes are not comfortable drinking during competition, or swallow large amounts of air, causing potential gastrointestinal distress. This can be remedied by practicing drinking during training. Many competitive distance runners find it best to slow to a walk and drink; the time lost is often made up through better performance due to proper hydration.

Despite the precautions, many long workouts and competitions result in dehydration despite fluid intake, since it is almost impossible to balance water loss. The stomach is only capable of emptying about 800 milliliters (26 ounces) of fluid per hour during vigorous activity, while water loss through sweating may be as high as 2 liters (68 ounces). Nonetheless, here are some general suggestions to consider:

- High amounts of sugar or its concentrated forms (glucose, sucrose or fructose) can reduce stomach emptying due to its high osmolality. A 10 percent glucose solution, for example, reduces gastric emptying by half.
- Older studies showed glucose polymers (maltodextrin) up to 7 to 8 percent may not slow gastric emptying, but others show the opposite effect, or no effect, depending on how the research was carried out.
- The ingestion of "glucose-polymer" drinks does not necessarily offer any advantage over regular glucose solutions in terms of metabolic or water balance.
- Small amounts of sodium may improve hydration, partly due to the fact that it can increase your thirst. The amount necessary can vary with athletes, but approximately one-third of a teaspoon of sea salt per liter may be a general guide.
- Fructose (as found in high-fructose corn syrup) may result in incomplete absorption and cause intestinal cramps or diarrhea, and may also result in malabsorption of iron, magnesium, calcium and zinc. In addition, fructose is converted much more slowly to blood glucose than plain glucose.

- L-glutamine may improve water, sodium, potassium and chloride absorption and may be useful during sports activities.
- The conflicts in the scientific literature probably indicate individual variations in athletes. Especially in the case of fluid replacement and electrolytes. Each person's needs must be considered independently. The best way to find out what works best for you regarding drinks and other nutrient intake during activity is to experiment during training (not racing).

Caffeine

Caffeine can have a significant impact on endurance. It is commonly used as an ergogenic aid, but often due to the presence of general fatigue. As such, many consume caffeine due to its drug qualities. Ask yourself if caffeine was decreased or eliminated, how it would affect your energy levels. If you're drinking it to keep your energy high, you're treating symptoms.

Caffeine is one of a group of compounds called methylxanthines, and is found in coffee, tea, chocolate, colas and a variety of over-the-counter drugs. The chart below lists the amounts of caffeine in some of these items. Amounts can vary significantly due to individual brewing methods, source, concentration, etc.

Intake of caffeine reaches peak concentration after about one hour and has an influence on the nervous, muscular and cardiovascular systems, with a resulting temporary increase in endurance. These improvements are most likely the result of increased utilization of fatty acids and sparing of glycogen. In studies, endurance increased equally (by 22 percent) with both relatively small and moderate amounts — 3 and 6 mg/kg doses, but higher doses of 9 mg/kg resulted in no further endurance, but the higher doses stimulated adrenal and nervous-system activity further. So relatively small amounts of caffeine can temporarily improve endurance. However, if you have increased adrenal stress, caffeine intake can further adversely affect your adrenals.

APPROXIMATE CAFFEINE CONTENT PER SERVING			
Brewed coffee	125-300 mg	Hot chocolate	25 mg
Instant coffee	90 mg	Green tea	less than 50 mg
Black tea	70 mg	Chocolate	45-55 mg
Cola	50 mg	Caffeine pills	15-280 mg

The ergogenic effects of caffeine are present with urinary caffeine levels that are below the limit of 12 micrograms/ml allowed by the International Olympic Committee. In addition to the potential legal issue, caffeine may pose health risks as noted, which could ultimately adversely affect performance. The most significant is dehydration; caffeine is a diuretic, and these effects may be amplified in hot weather and at altitude. Calcium and magnesium loss may be increased in those who consume caffeine, and caffeine may adversely affect bone metabolism, placing you at risk for bone loss or stress fractures. Immune function and the antioxidant system may also be adversely affected by caffeine intake. If you have excess adrenal stress, or problems with your immune or intestinal system, reductions or elimination of caffeine may be necessary.

Alcohol

Alcohol (ethanol) is generally not used as an ergogenic aid, but athletes consume more alcohol than non-athletes, so it's worth discussing its effects on human performance and health. Alcohol provides moderate amounts of energy (7 kcal/g). Moderate to large intakes may promote weight loss due to its substitution for carbohydrate, but this amount also inhibits fatty-acid oxidation, something which will also reduce your endurance.

Recent studies show mortality risk is greatest in those who abstain from alcohol, and those who consume more than two to three drinks per day, with the protective effect of moderate intake less in women. Most of this data reflects coronary disease risk. Alcohol in moderation may also have antioxidant effects. However, the risk of some cancers and liver stress may be elevated with moderate alcohol intake in some people. Higher alcohol intakes increase the requirements for various nutrients, including vitamin B1, folic acid, zinc and niacin. Like all other recommendations, light to moderate alcohol consumption is a very individual issue.

"Energy" Bars

There are dozens of so-called energy bars on the market. Unfortunately, most contain ingredients that are not healthy, containing very processed ingredients such as hydrogenated oils, high amounts of saturated fats, refined sugar (often disguised as maltodextrin or high-fructose corn syrup) or a combination of all. Most are also low in fiber. Many are made predominantly of high-glycemic carbohydrates, with little or virtually no protein or good fats. More important is the problem that many athletes use these imbalanced products as meals, and most bars do not qualify as a meal replacement since they are not made from real foods. Read labels. Very few bars would meet the healthy criteria outlined in this text. Use only products made from real food and avoid those containing high-glycemic and processed ingredients, especially those containing fats which interfere with the body's delicate eicosanoid balance. Phil's Bar meets this standard.

Healthy energy bars may be useful for athletes in a number of situations:

- As an in-between-meal snack, especially for those who should consume food every two to three hours (those with blood-sugar handling problems, adrenal stress and carbohydrate intolerance).
- As a healthy alternative to "junk-food" snacks or meals.
- As an easily accessible food when none is available; during work, school, travel, etc.
- During long training sessions or competitions.
- Following training or competition.

Another important use for bars containing carbohydrates, protein and fats is their ability to help replace glycogen stores. At one time it was thought that only glucose drinks were effective for replacing glycogen stores following a workout or competition. But it's now known that a mixed meal can also be very effective; a bar that contains complex carbohydrates, protein and good fat can fit this bill. The convenience of a bar allows you to immediately consume a healthy food, along with water, to accomplish this task.

While it is important to understand the current research, the athlete's needs are most important and may not always correlate with laboratory data. Through trial and error, you can find your optimal fluid and solid nutritional needs.

11

The Supplement Story

A nutritional supplement is just that — a product that supplements the diet rather than something that replaces part of the diet. It's important to try to meet all your nutritional needs from your diet — this should be a major focus when it comes to eating for endurance. For many reasons, you may not always be able to get all your nutrients from your diet. When you travel there is less control over what you eat, your work schedule may not be conducive to getting good food at each meal, our food supply may not be supplying all the appropriate needs due to soil depletion of nutrients, and other factors. If and when you can't get adequate nutrients from your diet, supplementing it can help ensure you meet all your nutritional needs — when it's done properly and with quality nutrients. Without the proper intake of these necessary nutrients, your endurance can be impaired.

This chapter addresses nutrition from a functional standpoint, rather than from the perspective of disease and preventing deficiency-diseases that are rare in industrialized countries. Nor does it give you a cookbook formula "this vitamin for that race distance." You may require specific nutrients to improve physical, chemical and mental/emotional function, even when blood tests are normal for these nutrients. The majority of athletes fall into the gap between overt deficiency and the levels of nutrient intake that allow optimal performance. Unfortunately, one key factor limiting efforts to determine athletic requirements for vitamin and mineral intake has been the unavailability of acceptable standards for evaluating the effects of marginal and mild deficiencies.

Taking nutritional supplements should be based on several factors. Most importantly, there should be some reasoning behind taking a specific product. This may be the result of a dietary analysis as discussed earlier, or as a trial basis based on various signs and symptoms, such as symptom surveys. Chapter 15 discusses various symptom surveys which may help you determine the best supplements for your needs. Beware of advertisements and other hype surrounding certain supplements; this should not be used as a basis for taking these products. Unfortunately, this is the most common reason people take certain products.

One of the most important recommendations regarding nutritional supplements should come from a professional. This should be done following a history, appropriate examinations, and sometimes blood, urine or other laboratory tests. Beware that professionals are not immune to marketing hype and sometimes take a shortcut and match a symptom with a supplement. For example, a patient who says fatigue is a problem may be given some iron pills. In addition, there is usually no one test that indicates a nutritional need, although in cases of anemia, for example, a simple blood test indicates low iron levels. But this does not, however, tell why the problem exists.

Nutrient Levels in Food

Individual nutrients may be adversely affected by a number of factors which reduce their levels in food. For example, many vitamins are unstable to the heat of cooking, including: vitamins A, C, thiamin (B1), riboflavin (B2), pyridoxine (B6) and E, biotin, the carotenoids (including beta carotene), folic acid and pantothenic acid (B5). In addition, lysine and threonine are amino acids unstable to heat. Also consider the following:

- During cooking, significant amounts of nutrient may be destroyed or lost in liquids if not consumed. For example, half the riboflavin (vitamin B2) in beef, up to half of the vitamin C in broccoli, and up to 60 percent of the riboflavin in spinach may be lost from overcooking.
- Compared to fresh foods, both freezing and canning results in lost nutrients. For example, niacin loss in frozen vegetables may be as high as 26 percent and in canned vegetables as high as 51 percent.
- Foods stored for longer periods may loose nutrients. After 48 hours, lettuce may lose 30-40 percent of its vitamin C content.

- Ripened foods generally have higher levels of nutrients. Tomatoes have more vitamin C and beta carotene when ripe compared to unripe; bananas have more vitamin C when ripe compared to medium-ripe or overripe.
- Vitamin E is destroyed by commercial cooking, food processing and deep-freezing.

Types of Supplements

There are three basic types of supplements available to people: natural food extracts, isolated products and synthetic products. Any one of these may have a place in your program, depending on your needs, although the first two are usually the best for most athletes.

Natural Supplements

Truly natural supplements are made from whole foods rather than just individual vitamins and minerals. These include products such as sesame seed oil (used to help reduce inflammation), collonsonia root (a natural herb useful for hemorrhoids), glandular products (such as dessicated liver or thymus) and other foods many athletes don't consume but that have such significant therapeutic actions that we may want to take them in supplement form: garlic, ginger or fenugreek are some examples.

Because they are made from foods, usually with the fiber and water removed, natural supplements contain most if not all the factors found in the whole food. While science has discovered some of the important individual substances necessary for optimal nutrition, such as certain common vitamins and minerals, it is very likely that many other important substances have not yet been discovered. Nonetheless, these undiscovered benefits are still available in food concentrates. Another example of these important nutritional substances are phytonutrients, which are found in whole foods.

Isolated Supplements

Isolated nutrients are another type of natural supplement, as they are derived from whole foods. Fish oil (EPA), for example, is made from fish. The fish-oil capsule contains only the oil and not the rest of the fish. L-glutamine is the amino acid as it is found in nature, but only this one isolated nutrient is used rather than the whole glutamine-rich food (such as meats, seeds and cabbage).

Other examples of isolated nutrients include specific vitamins and minerals that naturally occur in the same form as in foods. Some vitamins include thiamin (B1), riboflavin (B2), and folic acid. It's worth noting that natural isolated vitamins are in much lower doses compared to the high-dose synthetic versions. For example, in a large steak, a good source of thiamin, the total amount is less than 1 mg, whereas a synthetic tablet of B1 (thiamin hydrochloride) may be 25, 50 or even 100 mg.

Synthetic Supplements

Many vitamins can be synthesized chemically. These may resemble the natural version, but are not identical because in nature, other substances are associated with the particular nutrient. Vitamin C, for example, is found in nature alongside other substances — bioflavonoids and rutin to name just two — making it a whole complex. Without these other parts, vitamin C alone may not work as well as the natural complex.

In addition, minerals are often used in forms that do not occur in nature or may be difficult for the body to utilize. Dolomite, commonly used as a calcium supplement, is powdered rock — a form of calcium difficult, if not impossible, to digest and absorb. In addition, the efficiency of absorption of many minerals can be much lower than natural forms. Magnesium oxide, for example, is commonly used in fortified products because it is very cheap. However, the absorption rate of magnesium oxide is very low (18 percent) compared to more natural versions which may have absorption rates of 60 or 70 percent or higher.

As noted above, the dose of synthetic vitamins and minerals is usually very different — almost always much higher — than it occurs in nature. This may be a useful guide for you to differentiate between a synthetic or low-quality supplement, and a truly natural or higher quality product. Ascorbic acid (vitamin C), for example, is typically sold in 100, 500 or 1,000 mg doses. It would be difficult if not impossible to get this much vitamin C from a meal, or even a day's worth of meals. That's because the ascorbic acid used in these supplements is chemically made.

Also note the even amounts of individual synthetic nutrients found in the once-a-day type products. These may be in the form of dose, or percent RDA. This is a common example of marketing hype. The chart on the next page gives examples of how this can be portrayed on a label.

SUPPLEMENT MARKETING HYPE			
Dose-based		**Percent-based**	**% RDA:**
Vitamin A	20,000 IU	Vitamin A	100%
B1	50 mg	B1	100%
B2	50 mg	B2	100%
B6	50 mg	B6	100%
Niacin	50 mg	Niacin	100%
B12	500 mcg	B12	50%

Unfortunately, the synthetic nutrients are also those used to fortify many food products we buy — breads, cereals, bars, drinks, and many other packaged foods.

Nutrient Absorption

Once the right foods or supplements are taken, the ability of the body to digest and absorb them is an important issue. Even with optimal dietary intakes, if food is not first digested, and if the small intestine's absorptive mechanisms are not efficient enough to get the nutrients into the blood, nutritional imbalances can occur due to malabsorption. These problems are identical to those associated with not eating enough of the necessary nutrients. In other words, nutritional imbalances may be due to:

- Not consuming enough nutrients.
- Not digesting food or nutrients.
- Not absorbing the nutrients.

Two common causes of nutrient unavailability are dysfunction of the hydrochloric-acid mechanism in the stomach, which is a key step in the digestive process, and dysfunction of the small intestine's villi, the structure which actually absorbs nutrients.

Among the potential causes of poor digestion and absorption of nutrients is any type of stress, which may cause reduced production of hydrochloric acid in many individuals. This problem, along with other stress can also result in small-intestine dysfunction. Malabsorption, most likely from diminished hydrochloric-acid production, also increases with age. Reduced hydrochloric acid may also be the result of caloric restriction.

These problems can cause a relatively minor (compared to celiac disease) but clinically significant subclinical or functional malabsorption. This malabsorption syndrome can produce symptoms anywhere in the body — those subtle, nagging problems many people complain about, from headaches and stomach aches, to skin problems and fatigue. Many people who are not digesting efficiently do not have intestinal disease but more subtle indicators, such as excessive gas or stool odor. Many will not think to discuss these relatively minor intestinal problems, especially when their main complaints are more painful, such as low back pain.

Betaine hydrochloride is a supplement in tablet form that, when swallowed, is converted to hydrochloric acid in the stomach. Those under stress or who are not digesting properly may benefit from this supplement. The normal dose is two tablets after each meal. Betaine hydrochloride tablets should not be chewed when taken.

Dysfunction of the small intestine also can result in malabsorption. This problem is often due to reduced hydrochloric-acid production in the stomach, but other reasons as well. This includes any type of stress. The use of L-glutamine can be very useful in restoring small-intestine function and the normalization of nutrient absorption. The normal dose is between 500 and 1,000 mg taken in the morning and evening on an empty stomach with a large glass of water.

Adverse Reactions

Toxic reactions to excess vitamin and mineral supplements sometimes occur. These are usually the result of taking synthetic forms of nutrients rather than those naturally occurring in food concentrates of lower doses. Perhaps the most common adverse effect of supplementation is excess intake of iron. When the body has too much iron, it results in too much storage (as ferritin) which has been associated with an increased risk of heart disease and liver oxidative stress (free radicals).

Vitamin C can be toxic if given to a patient with excess iron (high ferritin levels) because of the potential oxidative stress posed by iron. This may also be true of those with excess copper. And too much niacin can impair aerobic function.

Excess intakes of vitamin D could produce imbalances, especially in athletes. This could result in disturbances with other nutrients, such as the essential fatty acids, which in turn can lower the amount of calcium entering your muscles and bones, and could result in muscle cramps and even weaker bones. Vitamin D is normally manufactured by the body, through the sun's action upon hitting our skin. Almost all athletes will meet more than their needs of vitamin D by training outdoors, even in the cold winter months. Taking extra vitamin D from supplements, especially considering vitamin D is used to fortify many foods, can result in an excess of this nutrient.

Excess amounts of vitamin A can also result in calcium loss from bones, predisposing one to stress fractures and those masters athletes to osteoporosis.

More common are the subtle problems associated with taking synthetic supplements. The more common harmful effect of taking nutritional supplements is the false sense of balance the athlete may derive; the belief that taking a once-a-day synthetic vitamin product, for example, may make up for the many imbalances in the diet.

Taking nutritional supplements may be a vital part of your endurance program. The key is to evaluate the need for specific nutrients that your diet is lacking through a diet analysis, completing a symptom survey to evaluate functional nutritional need, or through combinations of evaluations, especially with the help of a professional. Taking the truly natural supplements are the first choice since they are usually more effective and safer.

12

Supplementing Endurance

This chapter discusses some of the more important supplements that could have a major impact, directly or indirectly, on your endurance. Most nutrients will only work for you if your body is in need of them. For example, taking a lot of thiamin (vitamin B1), which is necessary to break down lactic acid, will not help you reduce lactic acid any quicker unless your thiamin levels are too low for your needs. In addition, it should be understood that specific vitamins don't give you more endurance. Instead, think of the balance of health and fitness, and that any vitamin deficiency can cause imbalances in your metabolism which can potentially have an adverse effect on endurance.

This chapter describes a variety of nutrients associated with specific endurance-related states and contains no "cookbook" remedies. For example, nutrients related to the aerobic system, those related to energy productions, and antioxidant nutrients, including those that support antioxidant activity are discussed. In addition, certain common nutrients are discussed since their actions are so different from what most people commonly believe, including the B vitamins, the E complex and others.

The Balance of Bs

Most of us are familiar with the B-complex vitamins. But what's most important about this group is the diversity in its actions. Rather than look at the B complex as one large group of vitamins, let's consider its functions. In this case, we can divide this complex into the "B" and "G" groups.

The B group consists mainly of thiamin, with other B-complex nutrients, and the G group contains predominantly riboflavin, along with other B-complex nutrients. The most common signs and symptoms associated with a potential need for B and G are listed below. Check off any symptoms you have to find out if you may benefit from either B or G.

GET THE RIGHT "B"	
Need for "B"	**Need for "G"**
❑ Carbohydrate intolerance	❑ Poor fat metabolism
❑ Sleepiness after meals	❑ Poor digestion
❑ Intolerant to noise	❑ Anxiety, excessive worrier
❑ Lack of vibration sense	❑ Restless/jumpy/shaky legs
❑ Frequent nighttime urination	❑ Whole body or limb jerks upon falling asleep
❑ Itchy skin	❑ Cracking at corners of mouth
❑ Decreased breath-holding time	❑ Rash on skin from shaving
❑ Frequent yawning or fatigue	❑ Very thin upper lip
❑ Decreased body temperature	❑ Burning or itchy eyes

Supplementing your diet with either the B or G part of the B complex can be done with products such as Cataplex B and Cataplex G, both made by Standard Process Inc. This is a natural food-based product which has a high-quality lower dose.

One unique feature of Cataplex B is the specific action of thiamin, which helps break down lactic acid produced, especially during anaerobic training and racing. Lactic acid reduces the function of muscles. It is released into the blood and quickly buffered to sodium (or potassium) lactate. This lactate is not a "waste" product as many people think, but is recycled in the liver to glucose and used for energy in the muscles. Studies show that people with low levels of thiamin have elevated lactate levels (along with low aerobic power and oxygen consumption).

A variety of studies have found high lactate levels to be associated with depression, anxiety, phobias and panic disorders, even in people with no psychiatric history. This correlates with the fact that increased dietary carbohydrates increase lactate production. Lower-carbohydrate diets, on the other hand, reduce lactate production.

Good sources of thiamin include meats, nuts, seeds, vegetables and whole grains (refining flour removes the thiamin, although some flour is enriched with it). This vitamin is unstable in oxygen and moisture, with significant losses in cooking and freezing.

Just as important to consider are the potential natural anti-thiamin substances found in nature, referred to as thiaminase. This enzyme can destroy thiamin, and is found in red chicory, Brussels sprouts, and red cabbage, with small amounts in tea. It is also contained in clams, oysters, squids and other mollusks and certain fish such as herring and smelt. This enzyme is easily destroyed by heat. Individuals who may have high needs for thiamin should consider avoiding these foods in their uncooked state.

As with many vitamins and minerals, some of the synthetic B vitamins can be harmful. For example, higher doses of niacin, as found in most synthetic vitamin products and fortified foods, can reduce aerobic performance. With the consumption of so much packaged and processed food today, and the indiscriminate use of synthetic multiple-vitamin products, many athletes take in large amounts of niacin, and other potentially harmful nutrients.

Supplementing with a large dose of thiamin may result in poor absorption. In addition to foods high in thiamin, when a supplement is used it's best to take a lower dose product, such as Cataplex B or G, taken three to four times daily as opposed to one high synthetic morning dose.

The Vitamin C Complex

Vitamin C is technically rated by the level of ascorbic acid in the supplement. Unfortunately, ascorbic acid, which is the antioxidant part of the vitamin, is only one piece of the vitamin C complex. Synthetically made ascorbic acid is nearly identical to natural form, except that all the other factors discussed below are not part of it.

In nature, there are other factors that make up this vitamin complex. Natural vitamin C complex supplements contain all the factors discussed below, without the very high dose of ascorbic acid. This is also more easily absorbed, whereas high-dose ascorbic acid is poorly absorbed. Other components in the vitamin-C complex are:

- The flavonoids, or bioflavonoids, also called vitamin P, are powerful antioxidants, and help strengthen blood vessels. Those who bruise easily or have bleeding gums may need more of the whole vitamin complex. These flavonoids, responsible for the colors in foods, are found in many vegetables, berries, citrus and other fruits, and red wine, and include phenols, rutin, hesperidin, quercetin, robinin and others.

- Vitamin K may also be considered part of the vitamin C complex. This is not only important for the normal clotting of blood (such as when you cut your finger), but is also necessary for the normal building and strengthening of bones. In this regard, vitamin K is at least as important a nutrient as calcium when it comes to bones. The best natural source of vitamin K is from the fat-soluble chlorophyll extract.
- Another part of the vitamin C complex is referred to as the J factor, which increases the oxygen-carrying capacity of the blood. Not much more is known about this factor.
- Tyrosinase is an important enzyme which is also part of this complex. It helps convert the amino acid tyrosine into thyroxin, an important thyroid hormone, and other chemicals necessary for good health and fitness.

Taking too much ascorbic acid can cause this vitamin to change from an antioxidant to a pro-oxidant, causing excess free-radical activity and inflammation. In addition, because ascorbic acid is a good acidifying substance (that may be one reason it's good for colds and other illness — some bacteria and viruses can't thrive in an acid environment), too much can cause excess acidity in the body. This can result in reduced ascorbic-acid absorption from the intestine. More serious may be that as ascorbic acid is increased, the body makes more ascorbase, an enzyme that breaks down ascorbic acid. It's possible that your body can destroy much of its vitamin C if you take large doses for long periods. Other side effects of ascorbic acid in high doses include the risk of kidney stones.

The Vitamin E Complex

There are two different types of vitamin E supplements: a very low dose that is all natural as a vitamin complex, that I'll call "vitamin E complex," and a high-dose vitamin E that only contains one part of the E complex — the tocopherols. Technically, vitamin E refers only to the tocopherols, and is rated by the amount of alpha tocopherol.

The low dose of vitamin E is found in food sources, usually only a few international units (IU) or less. This natural vitamin E complex includes the following makeup:

- Eight different tocopherols which act as antioxidants, including the important ones, alpha and gamma tocopherol.
- The phospholipids, an important part of cell-wall structures.
- Steroid hormone precursors important for hormone production.
- Essential fatty acids which were discussed earlier.

In foods, the amount of naturally occurring tocopherol is very small. For example, in a loaf of whole-wheat bread (which contains a relatively high level of natural vitamin E), only 2-4 IUs may be present.

Supplements that are great sources of natural vitamin E include wheat-germ-oil perles (which are sealed to keep oxygen from making the oil rancid), and Cataplex E (Standard Process), which also contains selenium, important for vitamin E activity. Selenium is an integral part of the antioxidant enzyme glutathione peroxidase. Supplementation of higher-dose synthetic vitamin E may also increase your need for additional selenium.

Separate from this vitamin source is the more traditional high dose of vitamin E, which is either an isolated or most often a synthetic source. This is made up only of tocopherols, and often only one type, alpha tocopherol, for example. The dose is typically 100, 200, 400 or even 800 IU. This type of vitamin E contains only tocopherol and the main action is that of an antioxidant. Although vitamin E, the generic name for all tocopherols, is labeled by the amount of alpha-tocopherol, high-dose products usually don't contain many, if any, of the other seven types of tocopherols as found in nature. Gamma-tocopherol, the most common form found in foods, is more effective in antioxidant effects than alpha-tocopherol, the most common isolated form in high-dose vitamin supplements. Large doses of synthetic alpha-tocopherol can displace gamma-tocopherol in the body. Gamma-tocopherol is also more effective in controlling oxidative stress in fats.

Taking too much synthetic vitamin E may lower thyroid hormone levels and slightly increase fasting triglyceride levels. High doses of vitamin E may also become pro-oxidants, acting in opposition to its normal antioxidant activity. This is more true with alpha-tocopherol, and less with gamma-tocopherol. In addition, high doses of vitamin E have been shown to cause muscle weakness, and may impair production of anti-inflammatory hormones.

Calcium-Magnesium Balance

Calcium supplements are still one of the hottest products on the market. Unfortunately, there may be more people with excess calcium than with true calcium deficiencies, despite what the advertising tells us. Many people have enough of this important mineral in their body, often due to large amounts taken from supplements, but are unable to put it to use. Poor calcium utilization, rather than deficiency, is almost at epidemic proportions. The end result of poor utilization may be the same as deficiency: not enough calcium gets into the bones and muscles where it is used, with the potential for calcium deposits in the joints or the kidneys as stones.

There are three important factors that enable us to use calcium:

- We must consume enough calcium-rich foods, and, if we don't, we must take an appropriate supplement.
- We must absorb the calcium in the foods we eat. The importance of nutrient absorption was previously discussed.
- After absorption, calcium must get into the cells of our bones and muscles (it's also used in other areas).

In general, smaller doses of calcium supplements are absorbed better than higher doses. For example, if you take a lower dose of calcium such as 300 mg, 70 percent may be absorbed, while a larger amount, such as 700 mg of calcium, may only have a 30-percent absorption rate. In both cases you absorb the same amount of calcium, 210 mg. So an important fact about calcium supplements is that it's best to take a lower dose several times a day rather than a large dose once daily.

The stomach's natural hydrochloric acid is also very important in making calcium more absorbable. Neutralizing stomach acid has a negative effect on calcium absorption, and a serious impact on digestion and absorption of all nutrients. Using antacid tablets as a calcium source may be the worst type of supplementation since it reduces natural stomach acid and results in malabsorption of calcium as well as many other nutrients.

Once calcium gets into the blood and is being carried to the muscles and bones, there is another important step to get calcium inside the cell. This calcium must be carried into the muscle and bone cells via a fat-dependent carrier, made from the A fat, GLA. Black currant seed oil contains high amounts of GLA and is very useful in getting calcium into the cells.

It's worth noting here that there are substances that can reduce calcium levels. Excess carbohydrates (too much fiber and phytic acid blocks calcium absorption), caffeine (reduces calcium levels in the blood) and phosphorus (pulls calcium out of bones and muscles) can be the most detrimental. Most soft drinks contain large amounts of phosphorus — and the kids who drink them also risk significant calcium loss from their teeth. Calcium is part of our complex chemical makeup. As such, it must be balanced with all other nutrients, especially magnesium. Too much calcium can cause a magnesium deficiency.

Magnesium helps our nerves, muscles and bones. This mineral is necessary for most enzymes to function, especially those important for energy production, to help control inflammation, and promote fat and sugar burning.

The magnesium content of our food supply may be diminishing. Excess sugar, vitamin D and stress can reduce our levels of magnesium. This combined with the fact that vegetables, the best source of magnesium, are not eaten in sufficient quantity by most athletes, makes supplementation of magnesium often necessary. When dietary analyses are performed, it is not unusual to see magnesium intake below RDA levels. Absorption of magnesium is best when it's in the form of lactate or citrate, and the worst form is magnesium oxide, which may be only 18 percent absorbable.

Choline

Choline is an essential nutrient. There are three important aspects of choline in relation to endurance. First, levels of this nutrient are reduced, sometimes significantly, by long training sessions or competitions lasting more than 90 minutes. Supplementing with choline can offset this reduction. Second, choline is the most effective natural remedy I have seen for those with asthma. Sometimes signs and symptoms of asthma are not obvious until exercise, when it is called exercise-induced asthma. Third, choline has anti-inflammatory effects. It may not be as powerful an action as balancing the A, B and C fats, but those athletes with inflammatory problems (tendinitis, fasciitis, arthritis and other conditions ending in "itis") generally need all the help they can get.

Doses of approximately 200 mg several times a day have been used successfully for asthmatics. In more severe cases, eight, ten or more tablets are used during the day for up to a month, followed by three to four tablets daily. The benefits of choline may be due to its beneficial effects on the nervous system, adrenal glands or a combination of both.

Choline can also be manufactured in the body from the amino acids serine and methionine, requiring vitamin B12 and folic acid.

Glandular Extracts

While the use of animal glandular products remains popular with many nutrition-oriented practitioners, very little scientific research has been conducted showing positive or negative effects of these supplements on humans. However, the clinical benefits of these glandular supplements continue to be observed. In mainstream medicine, the use of certain isolated substances from animals has proven effective for humans, such as bovine and porcine insulin, estrogen and other hormones. However, some practitioners have avoided the use of non-prescription nutritional animal supplements because of the lack of scientific evidence regarding their value.

These substances include products made from adrenal, pancreas, liver, thyroid, ovary, thymus and other glands. Other products are also used and produced from animal organs. In the wild, these animal parts are the first eaten by most predators, with much of the muscle meat left to scavengers. Overall, organs and glands have much more nutritional value. For example, liver averages 2.8, 7.5 and 71 micrograms/g of thiamin, pyridoxine and pantothenic acid, respectively; the same nutrients in muscle meat average 0.9, 3.3 and 4.7, respectively.

Thymus products are commonly used by complementary sports medicine practitioners, and are sometimes available in stores. Thymus and immune function is especially important in athletes since training can suppress this system. Human thymus function gradually diminishes with age, although it is still active in adults, and its loss of function can even be reversed. Thymomodulin, a calf-thymus derivative (composed of several peptides) has been used successfully for the treatment of food allergies and respiratory infections, and has been shown to regulate the maturation of human T cells.

Different types of preparations of the same gland are available, and used for different types of imbalances. Adrenal dysfunction for example, may be treated with the use of whole desiccated adrenal gland, or a glandular extract.

There are three types of glandular preparations:

- Aqueous tissue extracts.
- Whole glandular concentrates.
- So-called protomorphogens.

Aqueous tissue extracts are available as two main types; those containing hormones, and those that are hormone-free. The extracts which contain hormones are prescription items, and include thyroid, which contains the hormone thyroxine, and ovary, containing estrogen and progesterone. Their mode of action is clear; they are used as a hormone replacement for individuals whose ability to produce their own hormones is greatly diminished.

More common, however, is the use of non-prescription aqueous extracts which do not contain hormones. The reason for the beneficial actions is unknown. Common supplements in this category include thymus extracts which may be successful in improving the immune-system function. Others include ovary and prostate extracts.

Whole glandular extracts are dried, unprocessed products of individual glands, but do not contain hormones. They may be used when increased function is desired, but may be contraindicated when a gland is overactive. For example, during certain stages of adrenal stress, certain hormones are overproduced. In this situation, a whole adrenal concentrate may not be an appropriate choice. Rather, one of the other glandular preparations may be helpful. This supplement may function due to its content of raw materials needed by the organ or gland for balanced function, but this is speculation.

Protomorphogens are theoretically nucleoprotein extracts from the cells of specific organs and glands, and are used when there is either excess or deficient function. They may have actions that are antigen-like, interacting with circulating antibodies to specific organs or glands which may interfere with their repair process. Like whole extracts, protomorphogens do not contain hormones.

13

Antioxidants

It is now clear that anaerobic training and competition create increased oxidative stress. This is due to the production of oxygen free radicals. These chemicals can cause skeletal and muscle damage, inflammation, and can increase the aging process. Free radicals may be related to post-exercise muscle pain, disrupt our sodium/potassium regulation, and promote disease processes. (It should be noted that light and moderate training, however, can improve immune function by increasing the antioxidant activity.)

Here's a quick technical explanation: Free radicals are atoms or molecules containing one or more unpaired electron. When this free radical reacts with other non-radical molecules, a new free radical is created with the potential for a devastating chain reaction. When this occurs with the unsaturated fatty acids in cell membranes and lipoproteins, lipid peroxidation occurs.

Free-radical stress causes damage to LDL cholesterol, protein and DNA, and can adversely affect collagen and joint function, promoting joint dysfunction and ultimately disease.

Dietary antioxidants and supplements have a positive effect on "scavenging" these free radicals and may prevent much of the muscle damage associated with training and competition. The degree of free-radical damage may be associated with training intensity, with exhaustive workouts creating the most oxidative stress.

In addition to the exercise itself, being outdoors can also increase free-radical stress from air pollution and non-ionizing radiation (ultraviolet and microwaves). Excess intake and body stores of copper and iron may also be involved in the production of hydroxyl radicals, which can also have damaging effects. It should be noted that vitamin C can be toxic if taken with iron because of the potential oxidative stress posed by iron.

Antioxidant nutrients that have demonstrated benefits in reducing free radicals include vitamin E, selenium, and vitamin C (ascorbic acid). However, high doses of ascorbic acid may have a biphasic relationship between its concentration and effect, suggesting that an excess may have opposite effects compared to low doses, including the risk of kidney stones.

Other nutritional substances, not technically referred to as antioxidants, contribute to antioxidant defense. Glutathione, for example, has significant antioxidant activity, and consists of the amino acids cysteine, glutamic acid and glycine, and requires the mineral selenium for activation. Carotenoids are also antioxidants, as are flavonoids, originally called vitamin P by Szenti-Gyorgy who discovered them in 1936. These flavonoids, responsible for the colors in foods, are found in many vegetables, berries, citrus and other fruits, and red wine, and include phenols, rutin, hesperidin, quercetin, robinin and others. In addition, tumeric is a common spice which has significant antioxidant properties.

The so-called "age pigments" that can be observed in some people are usually end products of lipid peroxidation, indicating the potential need for more antioxidants.

Amino-Acid Supplementation

Supplementing the diet with amino acids is very common in the sports community; however, the research results have been mixed, with the exception of L-glutamine. The lack of extensive positive research with other amino acids may indicate the importance of individuality. I am always cautious about supplementing with individual amino acids due to the risk in worsening an amino-acid imbalance unless careful assessments are made. This may be less of a problem with L-glutamine which is utilized to a greater extent in the GI tract and is not completely absorbed. A number of studies on amino acids are of interest:

- Supplementing the diet with a complete protein source enhanced muscle-mass gains compared to subjects who trained without the supplement.
- Amino-acid supplements can lower cortisol levels in swimmers.

- Supplementing amino acids during endurance activities may improve negative protein balance and supplies substrate fuel.
- Male power athletes whose daily dietary protein levels were 1.26g/kg had serum amino-acid levels significantly lowered during intense training; leucine supplementation prevented the decrease in the serum leucine.
- Significant reductions in serum amino acids occur following very long workouts and races.

In addition to gastric function, small-intestine efficiency is also required for optimal nutrient absorption. L-glutamine is the primary fuel of the small intestine — more than sugar or fat — and this amino acid is vital for nutritional absorption. During stress, including training and competition, L-glutamine utilization increases dramatically. Doses of 500 mg to 2 g, two to four times daily between meals can help intestinal absorption of all nutrients.

Foods high in glutamine include meats and fish, seeds and sprouted seeds, and cabbage. However, even if glutamine is prevalent in the diet, significant amounts can be lost in food due to cooking as it is heat labile. In addition, avoidance of food (skipping meals, fasting, etc.), which can inhibit intestinal function, may further reduce glutamine levels; An extreme example is a four-day fast, which can reduce glutamine levels by 50 percent.

L-glutamine has been one of the most intensely studied nutrients in the field of nutrition in recent years. In addition to its use for intestinal stress and malabsorption, there are a number of other important aspects of L-glutamine to consider:

- L-glutamine improves water, sodium, and potassium absorption and may be useful during training and racing.
- L-glutamine has a positive effect on athletes' immune systems.
- L-glutamine supplementation following exercise may reduce infections.
- L-glutamine concentrations are decreased after long endurance training and racing.
- Overtraining is associated with reduced L-glutamine concentrations.

- L-glutamine has marked anti-inflammatory activity and moderate analgesic effects.
- L-glutamine also has positive effects on large-intestine function.

Nutrients Important for Carbohydrate Metabolism

As previously discussed, we get most of our energy from carbohydrates and fats. For this process to continue, however, a variety of nutrients are directly and indirectly essential. The most common ones are listed below:

- **Thiamin (B1)**
- **Pyridoxine (B6)**
- **Pantothenic acid (B5)**
- **Cobalamin (B12)**
- **Riboflavin (B2)**
- **Niacin (B3)**
- **Choline**
- **Biotin**
- **Chromium**
- **Magnesium**
- **Manganese**
- **Iron**

These nutrients are especially important for carbohydrate tolerance — the ability to metabolize this food group — and, low supply of any of these nutrients may adversely affect carbohydrate metabolism at various levels.

Low levels of chromium, for example, may contribute to the prevalence of glucose intolerance in the American and western-European populations, in part because this nutrient may be depleted through the refining of whole grains. Supplementing with chromium can improve carbohydrate tolerance. Chromium requirements may be higher during training. Consider other nutritional issues related to carbohydrate metabolism:

- Low levels of magnesium are associated with carbohydrate intolerance (CI).
- Zinc deficiency is associated with CI, and may be improved with zinc supplementation.
- Increased biotin intake can improve glucose dysfunction associated with CI. Raw egg whites, sometimes consumed by athletes, contain the glycoprotein avidin, which can bind biotin in the GI tract and prevent its absorption.
- Choline may help reverse insulin resistance.

In addition, fluoride can adversely affect carbohydrate metabolism (by blocking the enolase enzyme in the glycolysis pathway). The major source of this mineral for many individuals is from fluoridated drinking water and toothpaste, with tea and seafood containing smaller amounts. In addition, the use of oral contraceptives has a significant adverse effect on carbohydrate metabolism, more than doubling the risk of developing a deterioration in glucose tolerance compared to non-users.

Aerobic-System Nutrition

The aerobic muscle fibers derive their color from the high volume of blood vessels and especially the presence of myoglobin, a protein compound containing large amounts of iron. Myoglobin combines with oxygen released by the red blood cell, stores it and transports it to the mitochondria. This is a necessary function which promotes, among other actions, the utilization of fats for energy. Iron in hemoglobin is also important for delivery of oxygen.

Unfortunately, iron as a nutritional supplement has been heavily promoted in our society as a remedy for "increasing energy." There are many causes of fatigue, and regularly taking iron supplements may pose risks. The stored form of iron as ferritin in excess may be associated with an increased risk of heart disease, and can also increase free-radical production.

Evaluating the need for iron is best accomplished with a blood test which measures at least serum iron, hemoglobin and hematocrit, and ferritin. However, the need for iron may still exist even when blood levels are normal. A dietary analysis can determine whether your intake of this mineral is sufficient.

One of the most important aspects of the aerobic system is the mitochondria, the site of fat-burning (and a major site of antioxidant activity). This organelle is traditionally described as the "power house" of the cell, generating large amounts of energy for endurance. In order to achieve optimal mitochondrial function, various nutritional factors are necessary. These include the ones described above for the generation of energy.

Essentially, the macro- and micronutrients used by the aerobic muscle fiber and mitochondria are the same ones found in muscle foods — meat and fish. Carnitine is necessary for the transportation of fat to the mitochondria for fat-burning. Carnitine is available in the diet (mostly from meat) and can also be synthesized in the body from the amino acids lysine and methionine (this synthesis requires iron and vitamin C). Low dietary-protein intake may result not only in less carnitine intake, but less raw materials (lysine and methionine) to produce it, which may have adverse effects on fat-burning. Like other nutrients, muscle carnitine levels can be extremely low while the serum carnitine concentration is normal, making blood tests for this substance not conclusive. The use of L-carnitine supplementation may be helpful when levels are low.

Iron

Iron is an important nutrient for the aerobic muscles. As previously discussed, it's possible to have normal iron in the blood but too little in the muscle, causing the muscle to function improperly. Since the aerobic muscle primarily burns fat as a fuel, low muscle iron may adversely affect fat-burning. If supplements are necessary, a lower dose (i.e., up to 10 mg.) daily for a month or two may be enough. If you have a continuous need for iron, something more important may be missing. Taking iron for long periods, especially in large amounts, may be harmful.

Since the early 1980s, scientists have speculated about the important relationships between certain levels of stored iron and heart disease. Excess iron, even moderate amounts, may even prove to be a more significant risk factor for heart disease than cholesterol.

Iron is also important in the brain and nervous system; it aids in the production of neurotransmitters and other brain chemicals, and is in the protective covering of nerves. Iron is efficiently recycled in the body, with some loss occurring during exercise through sweating, or in menstruating women. Excess iron loss or decreased intake may produce a serious deficiency. On the other extreme, toxic amounts of iron may be deposited in the liver and spleen, resulting in cirrhosis of the liver or diabetes. Excess iron is also associated with certain neurological problems including Alzheimer's and Parkinson's disease, as well as multiple sclerosis.

When the body has enough iron for normal use, the remainder is stored in the form of ferritin. Recent evidence shows that ferritin may promote the formation of free radicals, which may injure cells lining the arteries and damage heart muscle as well as increase the level of LDL, the so-called "bad" cholesterol. Vitamin E's positive role in heart disease may be that it serves as an antioxidant, preventing excess free-radical formation and oxidative damage.

The marketing of iron to treat fatigue ("iron-poor, tired blood") may be one reason for excess accumulation of iron in some people. Almost all multiple-vitamin/mineral preparations contain too much of it, and many foods are fortified with iron. Certainly, if you are iron deficient, taking an iron supplement is necessary. But without knowing whether it's needed, iron supplementation should be avoided.

If a blood test for ferritin shows you have too much stored iron, the first thing to do is assess whether you are consuming too much. Often, excess iron stores are the result of an accumulation of iron over several years. In some situations, the body's metabolism may not be functioning properly, resulting in excess ferritin. Donating blood may be one way to help reduce excess iron stores.

14

The Two-Week Test

The Two-Week Test was developed many years ago in my practice to help the patient understand his or her specific dietary needs, especially for carbohydrates. This simple four-step test is performed over a two-week period. The goal is to reduce the body's production of insulin — a hormone which acts on glucose (from dietary carbohydrates). During this test, insulin levels remain relatively low because concentrated carbohydrates are not consumed.

There are four steps to the Two-Week Test:

1. Before the test begins, note symptoms which may indicate carbohydrate excess:

- ❑ Are you frequently or always hungry?
- ❑ Are you irritable or weak before meals or if meals are skipped?
- ❑ Do you frequently crave sweets?
- ❑ Do you often have feeling of depression, or are depressed?
- ❑ Do you get sleepy or experience reduced mental concentration following meals?
- ❑ Do you have intestinal bloating (gas) following meals?
- ❑ Does overeating carbohydrates or sweets make you feel bad?

- ❑ Do you avoid eating breakfast because it increases hunger during the day?
- ❑ Do the above symptoms improve with increased number of meals (i.e., five or six daily meals instead of two or three)?
- ❑ Do you have a history of oral contraceptive use?

It's important to write down these problems so that after the test you can objectively ascertain any improvements.

In addition, consider performing the MAF test as described in my book *Training for Endurance.* Your doctor or health-care professional may also want to perform other tests, such as vital capacity, blood pressure, triglyceride levels, and others. These (and any other) signs and symptoms can be used to assess the effects of the Two-Week Test.

2. For a period of two weeks, avoid eating all concentrated carbohydrate (high glycemic index) foods. These include:

- Bread, rolls, pasta, pancakes, cereal, muffins, rice cakes.
- All sweets, including all products that contain sugar (ketchup, honey, sports drinks and energy bars, and those in prepared foods (as indicated on the labels).
- Fruits and fruit juice.
- Potatoes (all types), corn, rice, beans.
- Milk, half-and-half, yogurt.

Foods that may be eaten during the Two Week Test, in unlimited amounts, include:

- Whole eggs, cheeses, cream, meats (beef, turkey, chicken, lamb, etc.), fish and shellfish. (Note that many processed and prepackaged meats have added sugar and should be avoided.)
- Tomato and V-8 juice.
- All cooked or raw vegetables (except potatoes and corn)
- Tofu.
- Nuts, seeds, nut butters.

- Oils, vinegar, mayonnaise, mustard, (no hydrogenated oils).

In addition, here are a number of important considerations:

- Prepare for this test by shopping for the foods required so they are readily available.
- Avoid becoming hungry between meals — unlimited smaller meals (i.e., snacks) of permitted foods may be necessary for some people and is encouraged. Those who eat four to eight smaller meals are usually not hungry.
- Do not worry about the volume of food being consumed, or potential imbalances of macronutrients — this will be balanced in the next step.
- Be consistent — performing the test for less than two weeks may not be a valid assessment unless there is an exacerbation of symptoms in which case the test should be ended.
- Consume enough vegetables (at least six servings per day) to maintain fiber intake and avoid constipation.
- Maintain a high volume of water intake.

3. After the Two-Week Test, re-evaluate the symptoms identified in your the initial assessment (in Step 1).

- If there were no changes (a negative test), or none that were significant, you may not be carbohydrate intolerant, and your previous level of carbohydrate intake may have been proper for your needs.
- If your symptoms improved (a positive test), this indicates your carbohydrate intake was previously too high. In some cases, a dramatic improvement is evident.
- If you feel worse following the two weeks it may be due to the drastic reduction of fiber, and usually indicates you did not consume enough vegetables. On occasion, a fiber supplement such as plain psyllium may be useful — but be sure to use a form that does not contain added sugar. This may be incorporated into the

diet at any time. Another possible reason you felt worse during the test would be that you became dehydrated. This may be possible because increased protein intake requires more water intake.

- If you performed a MAF test prior to the Two Week Test, repeat the MAF Test a week or two after the Two-Week Test ends. In many athletes, a significant improvement is attained in this second MAF Test.

4. If the Two-Week Test is positive, the next step is to determine how much carbohydrate you can tolerate without developing any of the symptoms that previously existed. This is accomplished as follows:

- Begin adding small amounts of carbohydrates to your diet. This may include one or two pieces of 100-percent whole-wheat toast with breakfast, some fresh fruit as a snack, or a small serving of brown rice with dinner. Continue to avoid sugar, processed carbohydrates and other high-glycemic foods.
- These added carbohydrates should not be eaten with consecutive meals, but only at every other meal during this process.
- After each addition, be alert for the return of any of the symptoms you had previous to the test. Especially note symptoms that develop immediately after eating, such as intestinal bloating, sleepiness, poor concentration or feelings of depression.

It is important to become aware of when, and if, your body has an adverse reaction to carbohydrate intake. By gradually adding more carbohydrates, you will generally find a level of intake that does not give you any adverse effects. This level may be significantly lower than the amount of carbohydrate you were previously consuming. At this point, it becomes much easier to find an optimal level of carbohydrate intake.

Once the level of carbohydrate intake is established, finding the proper levels of fat intake is accomplished by looking at the results of your dietary analysis and being sure that the ratio is corrected as necessary. This often involves adding certain fats to the diet, and removing others. Through this process, along with adjustments in carbohydrate intake, the amount of fat in the diet may be established. The same process is followed for protein. Typically, it may take several weeks to optimally balance macronutrients.

Body-Fat and Weight Loss

One measurement which may also be helpful is to weigh yourself before and after the two-week period. The specific purpose of this test is not to lose weight, but weight loss often occurs, even when the person eats more fat and calories. Studies have shown that this type of eating could produce significant body-fat loss within a two-week period.

Even better than stepping on the scale to measure your weight, is to measure your body fat. Body fat can not be measured on a scale because most of your weight is water and muscle, not fat. Calipers, immersion scales and other gadgets may be good averages of body-fat content but are no more consistent than if you simply measure your waist and hips.

Using a tape measure, check the circumference of your waist at the level of your belly button, and the measurement of your hips at the hip joint (the largest protrusion on the side of your pelvis area). Do this before starting the Two-Week Test, and afterwards. If you burn off body fat, you'll see these areas get smaller. And because fat takes up a lot of room but doesn't weigh much, you may see your waist and hips shrinking as you burn more body fat.

Not only is the waist and hip measurement a good index of fat loss, but an indication of potential future health problems. Heart disease, breast cancer, high blood pressure, stroke, diabetes, obesity and other health problems are associated with high measurements. Specifically, the ratio of the waist-to-hip measurements — determined by dividing the waist measurement by the hip measurement — is a predictor of future health problems. The ratio in men should be 0.8 or less, and in women 0.9 or less.

When you eat too many carbohydrates, much of it is converted and stored as fat, which takes up space, and also some water, which provides increased weight. After finding your optimal carbohydrate intake and maintaining it, your body fat and weight often are reduced — sometimes significantly. So weigh yourself before and after (but not during) the Two-Week Test. Any weight loss (above 3 pounds) is also an indication of a positive test.

15

Nutritional Symptom Survey

The usefulness of looking at all signs and symptoms the body creates rather than one particular symptom in one area can be an important form of assessment. Doctors frequently use this method, and studies have demonstrated its validity. The purpose of a symptom survey form is to help determine which nutrients may be beneficial.

Symptom surveys are best used in conjunction with other methods of evaluation, including a thorough history and physical examination. This chapter provides an inventory of many common symptoms that may reflect body dysfunction (as opposed to disease). It is this type of dysfunction that typically impairs endurance.

This symptom survey reflects dysfunction in a variety of areas. It is divided into groups based on certain very general physiological indicators. These groups have associated nutritional factors that, when taken regularly for a couple of months, can help improve function in this area. It should be noted that a number of these symptoms may appear in more than one group.

Take the symptom survey yourself, and let your family take it too. There are 10 groups. Check off the signs or symptoms you experience. First, read through and check off each box that applies to you. Then read about the possible related nutrients or dietary factors in the key after each group. These are only general guidelines. However, they can be very applicable and accurate for most athletes when it comes to matching the right supplements with the body's dysfunction. Compare these with other issues discussed earlier in this book.

I've also included the doses I recommended during my years in practice. I've had the most success with this when supplements are taken for at least two months, followed by a re-evaluation of the signs and symptoms. At that point, one of three issues will be evident:

- If there is partial improvement, continue for another two months, then re-evaluate again.
- If there is good improvement, stop the supplements and see if you can maintain good health (i.e., no return of the signs or symptoms) with just a good diet. If the problems return, begin the supplements again, and re-evaluate your diet to see if there are certain foods you should be including.
- If there is no improvement at all, you may have to re-evaluate whether you chose the right supplement(s), or possibly if you have a malabsorption problem (which may be helped by L-glutamine.

Group One

- ❑ Asthma, especially with exercise?
- ❑ Dry mouth, eyes, nose?
- ❑ Gag easily?
- ❑ Difficulty relaxing?
- ❑ Easily startled?
- ❑ Sensitive stomach?
- ❑ Appetite reduced?
- ❑ Hands and feet cold and clammy?
- ❑ Keyed up?
- ❑ Intolerant to acid foods?

Group Two

- ❑ Joint stiffness in morning?
- ❑ History of kidney stones?
- ❑ Eyes or nose watery?
- ❑ Perspire easily?
- ❑ Constipation-diarrhea alternating?
- ❑ Hoarseness in throat?
- ❑ Rapid digestion?
- ❑ Muscle cramps at night?

- ❏ Eyelids swollen or puffy?
- ❏ Digestion rapid/hungry often?

Groups One and Two are related to the nervous system. The sympathetic part revs you up for a race, increases your muscle power, and is your fight-flight mechanism. The parasympathetic part calms you down, allows you to eat a meal, and relax. However, sometimes there is too much of one or not enough of the other. For example, if you're trying to get up for a race but your sympathetics are not stimulated enough, you won't race as well. Or, if you're trying to relax at dinner but your sympathetics are too active, you won't digest your food as well.

Group One symptoms may be associated with excess sympathetic or diminished parasympathetic function. Nutrients commonly used to help remedy this imbalance are choline, potassium and magnesium. The dose for choline is typically about 200 mg three times daily (more if you have asthma), and a product called Organic Minerals (for potassium and magnesium), one tablet three times daily.

Group Two symptoms may be associated with excess parasympathetic or diminished sympathetic function. The most common nutrient used to help remedy this imbalance is phosphorus, usually in the form of the supplement of liquid phosphoric acid. I typically have used 10 drops of Phosfood in water after each meal.

Group Three

- ❏ Chronic fatigue?
- ❏ Dizziness upon standing?
- ❏ Crave salt?
- ❏ Allergy or asthma?
- ❏ Low back, knee or ankle problems?
- ❏ Low blood pressure?
- ❏ Nails weak or ridged?
- ❏ Insomnia?
- ❏ Sensitive to bright light?
- ❏ Sexual desire reduced?

Group Three is associated with adrenal-gland dysfunction. When considering adrenal problems, it's important to determine which hormones are produced in excess, and which are lacking. A general supplement very useful for those with adrenal stress is L-glutamine, because the small intestine is usually less efficient in its absorptive capabilities — so typically, other nutrients may be malabsorbed. I typically have used 500-1000 mg morning and evening on an empty stomach with a large glass of water.

Group Four

- ❑ Indigestion two to four hours after meals
- ❑ Rheumatoid arthritis
- ❑ Chronic anemia
- ❑ Loss of appetite (especially for meat)
- ❑ Coated tongue
- ❑ Foul-smelling gas
- ❑ Intestinal disease
- ❑ Over age 60
- ❑ Calorie restriction often
- ❑ Recurrent yeast or fungal infections (i.e., candida)

Group Four is associated with poor stomach function, specifically reduced hydrochloric acid. This may also be common in those under stress. Betaine hydrochloride tablets (which turn to the same hydrochloric acid your stomach makes) can be taken when needed for a couple of months. After this time, your stomach may be more capable of making its own hydrochloric acid, although some people require this supplement for much longer periods. Two tablets after each meal is the typical dose, or one tablet after a snack.

Group Five

- ❑ Sleepy after meals
- ❑ Bloated after meals
- ❑ Poor concentration after meals
- ❑ Always hungry
- ❑ Increasing abdominal fat and/or facial fat (cheeks)
- ❑ High waist-to-hip ratio
- ❑ Fingers swollen/tight after exercise
- ❑ Diabetes (or in family)
- ❑ High blood pressure, cholesterol or triglycerides (or in family)
- ❑ Heart disease, stroke, breast cancer (or in family)

Group Five is associated with carbohydrate intolerance (CI). This common problem was discussed in Chapter 7. The nutrients I most commonly suggest for those with this problem include the omega-3 fats, fish oil or flaxseed oil — two capsules after each meal. These are often needed regularly unless your diet contains enough of these hard-to-get fats. Certain minerals are also commonly needed: chromium, magnesium and zinc. Smaller doses of these three times daily are better than one large dose.

Group Six

- ❑ Aspirin (or other NSAIDs) improves symptoms
- ❑ Chronic inflammation
- ❑ Menstrual cramps
- ❑ Dry itchy skin or scalp
- ❑ Overeating sweets or high carbohydrates upsets
- ❑ Eat in restaurant, take-out or fast food often
- ❑ Seasonal allergies
- ❑ Low-fat diet
- ❑ Depression
- ❑ History of tumors or cancers?

Group Six is associated with essential fatty-acid imbalance. This issue was addressed in Chapter 4. The only effective way to balance your fat is to evaluate your diet, which will determine your omega-6 and -3 ratio. If these fats are not balanced, reduce the excess and supplement with the fats that are lacking. Most often, it's the omega-3s that are too low, with too much omega-6. As previously discussed, other nutrients may also be important, the most common being vitamin B6, niacin, and magnesium.

Group Seven

- ❑ Carbohydrate intolerance
- ❑ Intolerant to noise
- ❑ Lack of vibration sense
- ❑ Frequent nighttime urination
- ❑ Itchy skin
- ❑ Decreased breath-holding time
- ❑ Frequent yawning or fatigue
- ❑ Decreased body temperature

- ❑ Sleepiness after meals
- ❑ Low blood pressure

Group Eight

- ❑ Poor fat regulation
- ❑ Poor digestion
- ❑ Anxiety
- ❑ Restless, jumpy, shaky legs
- ❑ Body or limbs jerk upon falling asleep
- ❑ Cracking at corners of mouth
- ❑ Rash on skin from shaving
- ❑ Thinning upper lip
- ❑ Burning or itchy eyes
- ❑ High blood pressure

Group Seven and Eight refer to the need for different parts of the B complex vitamins. This was discussed fully in Chapter 12.

Group Nine — Children Only

- ❑ Low birth weight (less than 5.5 pounds)
- ❑ Taller than average for age
- ❑ Increased weight or body fat
- ❑ Sleep problems
- ❑ Mother: increased stress during pregnancy
- ❑ Increased aggression or anger
- ❑ Hyperactive
- ❑ Attention Deficit Disorder (ADD)
- ❑ Overeating sweets or carbohydrates upsets
- ❑ Athletic activity low

Group Nine is associated with signs and symptoms in kids that may indicate poor carbohydrate metabolism. The same nutrients would apply, but using half the dose, as discussed in Group Five.

Group Ten

- ❑ Eating breakfast increases hunger all day
- ❑ Eat "energy" bars often

- ❑ Frequent hunger
- ❑ Low blood sugar
- ❑ Sleepy after meals
- ❑ Skip meals often
- ❑ Insomnia
- ❑ Irritable/shaky if meals are delayed
- ❑ Crave candy in afternoon or evening
- ❑ Eat junk food often

Group Ten is a list of signs and symptoms common in people who could benefit from eating healthy snacks. These snacks should be made from real food, like Phil's Bar, or save some of your breakfast or lunch for a snack two or three hours later. Snacking can increase fat-burning, reduce weight and improve other areas of your metabolism (such as reducing insulin and cholesterol, and stabilizing blood sugar).

16

Diet, Nutrition and Overtraining

Overtraining is a common problem in athletes. I would estimate about half the new patient athletes I saw in practice were overtrained. However, many of these athletes would not readily admit that they had a problem. Overtraining is not a well-defined syndrome, and most athletes think that the typically overtrained individual is broken down, burned out and unable to perform. Certainly this is true of the chronically overtrained athlete. However, early stages of overtraining are more subtle. (For more detail on the overtraining syndrome see my book, "Training for Endurance").

Unfortunately, many athletes who are well on their way to being overtrained continue at their normal or near-normal levels of training. Eventually, performance declines, energy is diminished and overall health is reduced. This section lists some of the commonly needed dietary and nutritional aspects observed in overtrained athletes from the earliest stage of this problem. Obviously, the causes of overtraining must be found and corrected.

While no overtraining protocol exists, certain common factors are related to overtraining. The most common problem is malabsorption of nutrients from the small intestine. The increased sympathetic stress causes reduced function in the small intestines. Malabsorption can begin a series of secondary nutrition problems. Betaine hydrochloride can improve digestion and nutrient absorption in those who are overtrained by increasing acid in the digestive system.

Overtrained athletes often experience a decreased plasma glutamine concentration, especially after each endurance training session or competition. Low glutamine levels are associated not only with reduced immunity, the reason overtrained athletes are often sick, but also malabsorption. L-glutamine supplementation can help improve both immune-system and small-intestine function.

Not only can what you eat have an impact on overtraining, but lifestyle issues can also play a role. Eating while driving or working, for example, adversely affects digestion and nutrient absorption.

Caffeine consumption may be contraindicated for overtrained athletes. Reduction or avoidance of stimulants such as coffee, tea, and soda, as well as caffeine-containing over-the-counter and prescription drugs, may be necessary.

Overtraining may disrupt the normal balance of eicosanoids, which balances the inflammatory and anti-inflammatory state. Careful evaluation of your diet, with particular attention to the ratio of fats, is vital. Omega-3 supplementation is most often necessary.

Zinc and phosphorylated serine may help reduce the abnormally high levels of cortisol common to overtrained athletes. This may especially be important if you wake in the middle of the night unable to easily get back to sleep. In this case, take these supplements just before going to sleep, and another as soon as you awaken during the night.

Reduction of high-glycemic foods, and eating smaller, more-frequent meals can greatly help overtrained athletes. These two steps can help to counteract the abnormally high cortisol found in most overtrained athletes, especially those who have symptoms of depression, which are also common during overtraining. Moderating carbohydrate intake may also be helpful as higher-carbohydrate diets may further elevate cortisol levels. An inadequate caloric intake and eating disorders may also exist with overtraining, and these can further adversely affect hormone imbalance.

Some overtrained athletes need additional choline. This is almost always the case when overtraining is associated with asthma, or so-called exercise-induced asthma. Recurrent asthma symptoms may be an early symptom of overtraining and usually respond well to choline supplementation.

17

Not for Women Only

Women possess a potential natural superiority to men in endurance sports through their greater capacity to burn fat. Since fat-burning is one of the keys to success in endurance sports, eating and training to develop maximum fat-burning may give women an edge.

Unfortunately, women are just as vulnerable as men to messing up body structure, chemistry and mental state. One of the significant problems frequently seen in women athletes, but not uncommon in men, is hormonal imbalance. This is influenced not only by training, but also to a larger degree by diet and nutrition.

One of the most obvious feminine problems resulting from imbalances in diet, nutrition and training is menstrual problems. Menstrual dysfunction comes in many forms, including amenorrhea (the absence of menstrual bleeding), oligomenorrhoea (a menstrual cycle between 35 and 90 days), and delayed menarche. So-called premenstrual syndrome (PMS) and menopausal problems are also common complaints by endurance women. There is no clear single cause and effect between menstrual dysfunction and training, diet, nutrition or other factors not reviewed here (including psychiatric factors). However, hormonal imbalance is a common denominator. Menstrual problems, and accompanying hormonal imbalance, are frequently associated with overtraining, especially when high-intensity training has been performed. Various diet and nutritional factors also can be a significant factor, as discussed below.

Amenorrhea is the most common menstrual problem affecting female endurance athletes. This problem may occur at a very early age. In a study of high-level athletes only 40 percent of runners (average age 13.6 years) had started menstruating compared with 95 percent of non-competitive girls of a similar age.

The problems in many amenorrheic athletes may be considered part of a syndrome, comprising overtraining (too much training volume and/or intensity) and disordered eating (especially reduced kilocalorie intake and excessively low fat intake). In addition, excessively low body weight and/or body fat (especially femoral fat stores: fat around the hips, buttocks and thighs), and vegetarianism can pose problems.

One of the most significant structural problems associated with amenorrhea is bone loss. Prolonged low estrogen and progesterone levels that accompany this problem increase the risk of decreased bone density, stress fractures, muscle soreness and physical fatigue. Demineralization of bone is most common in the spine, wrist and metatarsals. These imbalances can lead to structural problems in the skeleton later in life due to osteoporosis. In addition, scoliosis is also associated with amenorrhea in athletes. (It should be noted that men can also have reduced hormones, specifically testosterone, which adversely affects bone density, also causing bone loss.)

The hormonal imbalance associated with amenorrhea and other hormonal problems is usually associated with adrenal-gland dysfunction, resulting in adrenal-hormone imbalance. Cortisol, a key adrenal hormone, is frequently elevated in amenorrheic athletes, as is the case in many overtrained athletes. Elevated cortisol is associated with reduced DHEA, another important hormone, which is associated with diminished estrogen and progesterone which in turn adversely affects the menstrual cycle. The reduced estrogen and progesterone profiles typical in amenorrheic athletes are actually very similar to those of postmenopausal women. These and other hormones, such as testosterone, are easily measured in athletes, as is discussed below.

In many cases, amenorrheic athletes consume an energy-deficient diet. Laughlin and Yen (in the *Journal of Clinical Endocrinology and Metabolism*, 1996) state, "growing evidence suggests that menstrual disturbances in female athletes are related to the metabolic cost of high levels of energy expenditure without compensatory increases in dietary intake." In some cases, however, amenorrheic athletes consume the same total kilocalories as those with normal menstrual cycles, but much less fat (up to 50 percent less) and less protein, with higher carbohydrate intakes. Reduced fat intake can result in lower intakes of essential fatty acids that can result in lower calcium absorption and lower bone calcium. This is typically aggravated by low dietary-calcium intake. Low calcium levels in the body can exist even when blood tests show normal blood calcium levels. We all need more than calcium for strong bones. Many other minerals, including magnesium, sodium and manganese are important. But more important — even more important than calcium itself — is vitamin K. I've used a natural vitamin K made from fat-soluble chlorophyll (Chlorophyll Complex) for patients who needed to improve bone health.

Disordered eating itself is a complex mental/emotional issue and a full spectrum of problems ranging from functional to pathological; i.e., from poor eating, dieting and preoccupation with low-fat, to clinically diagnosed anorexia nervosa and bulimia (a discussion of which goes beyond the scope of this book).

Amenorrhea and other menstrual problems in many athletes is often thought of as having psychogenic origins, but it has been shown that nutrition and hormonal imbalance can be more of a cause. The important relationship between training and nutritional imbalance is best remedied conservatively to re-establish normal hormonal profiles and menstrual activity in amenorrheic athletes, including the use of natural hormones.

In athletes without amenorrhea, other menstrual distress such as PMS is still common and also frequently associated with increased consumption of carbohydrates and depression. Also, menstrual problems are often accompanied by reduced immune function, causing women to be more vulnerable to any type of infection — from bacteria and viral, to yeast and fungal infections (i.e., Candida). Infertility is also a problem for some women and is mostly due to hormone imbalance and carbohydrate intolerance.

In postmenopausal women, estrogens may not be made in sufficient amounts in the adrenal glands, but DHEA production can make up for this since it is a precursor of estrogen. The end result is that a healthy postmenopausal women should make enough estrogen from DHEA. In addition, some testosterone is converted to estrogen (estradiol), and DHEA can be converted to testosterone via androstenedione.

The ABCs of Hormones

Our hormones are typically produced from the head down, by glands throughout the body (some hormones are made in organs such as the heart and intestines). Generally, the process starts in the brain. A common scenario may be as follows: The hypothalmus is next to and communicates with the area in our brain that controls emotions. The hypothalmus produces specific hormones that affect the pituitary, which sends its hormone, ACTH (adrenocorticotropic hormone), down to the body where certain glands (i.e., the adrenals) are stimulated to produce its hormones. This is referred to as the hypothalmic-pituitary-adrenal axis. Another important connection is the hypothalmic-pituitary-ovarian axis, which is critical in estrogen and progesterone production. The hormones in each of these mechanisms can affect the other mechanisms. Virtually any hormone, emotion or stress can affect any other hormone. This gives you an idea of how complex things can get.

Hormone production by specific glands comes and goes as needed. The most important function is to help control stress, body development, repair and growth (such as muscles and bones), and sexual function. They also help us burn sugar and fat for energy, regulate electrolytes and water, and help get us through the day, a workout or race. When a disruption in the balance of hormones takes place, problems can occur in the form of dysfunction, pro-

HORMONES AND THE GLANDS THAT MAKE THEM

Hormone	Chief production site
Cortisol	adrenals
DHEA	adrenals
Testosterone	adrenals, ovaries, testes[1]
Estrogens[2]	ovaries (small amounts from adrenals)[3]
Progesterone[4]	ovaries (small amounts from adrenals)
Insulin	pancreas

1. Both men and women make all three sex hormones — estrogen, progesterone and testosterone. The difference between genders is amounts; women make more estrogen and progesterone, and men make more testosterone.
2. The three major estrogens include estriol, estradiol and estrone.
3. In men, some testosterone can be converted to estrogen.
4. Progesterone can be converted to estrogen and testosterone.

ducing signs and symptoms. For example, reduced levels of estrogen and progesterone can result in amenorrhea; in both males and females, low testosterone can impair recovery from workouts and races and reduce sexual desire. These are common problems in many athletes, along with reduced DHEA. Excess cortisol is often a primary problem (and sometimes excess insulin production as well).

The most common problem when adrenal stress and hormone imbalance occurs is an excess level of cortisol and reduced DHEA, resulting in an anabolic/catabolic imbalance.

As we train and race, we must rebuild our bodies — especially the muscles, but also bones, blood vessels, the heart and immune system. This is referred to as being in an anabolic state. When the body is breaking down, it is referred to as a catabolic state. This tearing-down process takes place as part of the training cycle, but too much catabolic activity leads to injury, ill health and reduced performance — the overtraining syndrome.

The right balance of anabolic and catabolic activity is necessary in order to reach athletic potential, without overtraining. In addition to high cortisol and low DHEA, low testosterone in both men and women is associated with an anabolic/catabolic imbalance.

High cortisol and low DHEA can be associated with:

- Reduced fat-burning and increased reliance on sugar.
- Increased insulin levels.
- The potential for more unstable blood-sugar problems.
- Bone loss.
- Calcium deposits (joints, blood vessels).
- Reduced immunity (increased infections).
- Reduced testosterone.
- Amenorrhea.
- Reduced reproductive status/fertility (men and women).
- Overtraining.

- Lowered breathing efficiency.
- Reduced sodium and water levels (adding to potential dehydration and hyponatremia).
- Training- and racing-associated diarrhea.

Recall that increased stress of any type can raise cortisol, especially anaerobic training.

DHEA supplementation has become very popular with athletes in recent years, with this product now available over the counter. Under high levels of chronic stress, including intense exercise, DHEA levels are often reduced as cortisol rises. DHEA also diminishes with age, with the highest levels occurring between ages 20 and 30, followed by a 10 percent decline each decade. With reduced DHEA, lower levels of testosterone and estrogen follow: DHEA contributes to about half the circulating testosterone in men, and in women DHEA may contribute to 100 percent of the estrogens.

Like high cortisol, reduced DHEA is an indication of potential overtraining and/or chronic stress. In addition, insulin levels above normal can further suppress DHEA production. DHEA supplementation, however, lowers insulin levels and increases testosterone in both men and women.

Hormonal Symptom Survey

When hormone imbalance occurs, it's not unusual for the athlete to have a variety of seemingly subtle symptoms, although often they are more dramatic. Sometimes it's the subtle symptoms that provide you with early clues of hormone imbalance. If you can "read" your body, correction of these imbalances as early as possible prevents more significant problems later. On the next page is a seven-part symptom survey that pertains to common complaints associated with hormone imbalance. Check off each item that pertains to you, and then read the general indications following the survey. If you have two or more of these symptoms, it may indicate a problem in this category, with more symptoms often associated with more severe imbalance. This may help you determine which hormones may be too high or too low, and is the first step to effectively correcting the imbalance. Ask yourself if you have any of the following:

Symptom Survey No. 1

- ❑ Chronic fatigue?
- ❑ Dizziness upon standing?
- ❑ Crave salt?
- ❑ Allergy or asthma?
- ❑ Low-back, knee or ankle problems?
- ❑ Low blood pressure?
- ❑ Nails weak or ridged?
- ❑ Insomnia?
- ❑ Sensitive to bright light?
- ❑ Sexual desire reduced?

General adrenal dysfunction. This is usually associated with high cortisol and low DHEA (followed by low testosterone, estrogen and progesterone), although other patterns can occur. In chronic stress and overtraining, for example, all hormones are low. Evaluating the other symptom-survey groups can help find a more precise pattern of imbalance, which is important to know before attempting to remedy the problem.

Symptom Survey No. 2

- ❑ Increased body fat/weight?
- ❑ Chronic fatigue?
- ❑ Slow metabolism?
- ❑ Below-normal (98.6 degrees F) body temperature?
- ❑ Sensitive to cold?
- ❑ Cold hands and feet?
- ❑ Skin dry or scaly?
- ❑ Hair coarse, hard to manage or falling out?
- ❑ Reduced initiative?
- ❑ Sleepy during day?

Low thyroid function. Most underactive-thyroid problems are referred to as "subclinical" and are without abnormal blood tests. Low oral temperatures (below 98.6 degrees F) may be an indicator of low thyroid activity. In many cases, thyroid dysfunction is secondary to adrenal-hormone imbalance. Certain nutrients, such as iodine, essential fats and natural progesterone cream may be helpful.

Symptom Survey No. 3

- ❑ History of bone fractures?
- ❑ Low bone density?
- ❑ Poor recovery from workouts?
- ❑ Lack of sexual desire?
- ❑ Overtrained?
- ❑ Poor muscle development?
- ❑ Use of tetracycline?
- ❑ Low-fat diet (current or previous)?
- ❑ Low-cholesterol diet (current or previous)?

Low testosterone levels. This is usually secondary to low progesterone and/or low DHEA. It can improve with natural progesterone cream in both men and women, and sometimes DHEA if carefully monitored (*Do not* take DHEA for more than one to two months).

Symptom Survey No. 4

- ❑ Depression
- ❑ Amenorrhea
- ❑ Poor recovery from racing
- ❑ Frequent hunger/cravings
- ❑ Increased fat in face or abdomen
- ❑ High insulin levels
- ❑ Low DHEA
- ❑ Frequent high-intensity workouts (including weight-lifting)
- ❑ Reduced immunity (increased colds, flu, asthma, infections, etc.)
- ❑ Easy to get to sleep but waken in middle of the night?
- ❑ Reduced fat-burning?

High cortisol. This is the most common adrenal-hormone problem. When elevated, other hormones of the adrenals are reduced, especially DHEA, testosterone and estrogen. The most common nutrients used to lower cortisol include zinc and phosphorylated serine. Lifestyle factors, such as overtraining and any other stress must be addressed (see *In Fitness and In Health* or *Training for Endurance*).

Symptom Survey No. 5

- ❑ Over age 40?
- ❑ Low testosterone?
- ❑ Low estrogen?
- ❑ High cortisol?
- ❑ Chronic stress?
- ❑ Regular hard exercise (including weight-lifting)
- ❑ High insulin levels?
- ❑ Low sodium during long training?
- ❑ Poor hydration?
- ❑ Overtrained?

Low DHEA. This is usually secondary to high cortisol, and therefore addressing this primary problem is a key to successful management. DHEA supplementation should be limited to one or two months if used at all.

Symptom Survey No. 6

- ❑ Water retention/edema?
- ❑ Reduced sex drive?
- ❑ Low blood sugar?
- ❑ Cravings for sweets?
- ❑ Increased body fat/weight?
- ❑ Swollen/painful breasts?
- ❑ Depression
- ❑ Mood swings
- ❑ Heavy or irregular menses
- ❑ Uterine fibroids

Excess estrogen. If this is due to estrogen replacement, your doctor may have to modify your dose or use a different type of estrogen if necessary. Vitamin B1 and B6 may also be necessary as these nutrients are often lowered with estrogen therapy.

Symptom Survey No. 7

- ❑ Fluid retention
- ❑ Low estrogen or testosterone
- ❑ History of breast cancer

- ❑ History of miscarriage
- ❑ Inflammatory problems
- ❑ Blood-sugar problems
- ❑ Reduced sex drive
- ❑ History of stress fracture or osteoporosis
- ❑ Reduced fat-burning (increased body fat)
- ❑ Low body temperature (below 98.6 degrees F)

Low progesterone. This is often the result of excess production of cortisol. The use of natural progesterone cream can be very effective, along with lifestyle modifications (i.e., stress reduction, including reduced anaerobic training).

Measuring your Hormones

It is easy to measure the levels of cortisol, DHEA, estrogen, progesterone and testosterone in athletes. This provides you with a more precise indication of which hormones are not balanced. A retest after a few months of improved diet, nutrition and training also ensures you're heading the right direction toward better health and fitness. This test is done by measuring the specific hormone levels contained in your saliva, rather than performing the test using blood. In addition to being more convenient and less expensive, salivary tests can also be more accurate than a blood test.

Natural Remedies

Once you have determined you have a hormone imbalance, a variety of natural therapies may be useful. The key is finding the remedies that best match your particular needs. Once you perform the hormone tests, and take the symptom surveys you will have a much better idea which hormones are too high, too low or just right.

Below are some natural remedies which can help correct hormone imbalances. You may have to consult with a professional for more individualized care, or for certain natural hormones only available by prescription.

Nutritional Factors

Almost any nutrient in low levels can have a negative impact on your hormonal status. Performing a nutritional dietary assessment is often a vital evaluation if you want to truly correct hormone imbalance. This will help you determine what, if any, nutrients are low (or excessively high) so you can immediately solve that problem.

High cortisol is a common problem, and there are a variety of nutritional factors that can help:

- A dose of 25 mg of zinc can reduce adrenal cortisol output significantly. Taking zinc two to four hours before your high cortisol period(s), as determined from your saliva test, may be the most successful remedy for this problem. Or, if you have high cortisol throughout the day and evening, take small amounts of zinc (10 mg) four times per day. Chewing the zinc may help its utilization. Foods high in zinc include protein foods such as meats, fish and eggs, oatmeal and seeds. Diets high in grains (breads, cereals) contain large amounts of phytates that may impair zinc absorption, as well as absorption of other minerals such as iron, calcium and magnesium.

- Phosphorylated serine or phosphatidylserine can be very helpful in reducing high cortisol. Phosphorylated serine, 100 mg three to four times daily, may be a good starting point, and used for three months. If cortisol levels are normal at this point, stop taking the supplement. If cortisol is not yet normal, use a different version of the supplement, phosphatidylserine, at the same dose for another three to six months and then retest. (Note that if your calcium intake is low, it's important to take additional calcium when taking either of these supplements due to its high phosphorous content.)

- Secondary to the above two nutrients, pantothenic acid, vitamin B6 and vitamin C may also be of general help for adrenal function. Dosages vary with individuals, but avoid high amounts: 100 mg of vitamin C one to two times daily, 100 mg of pantothenic acid one to three times daily, and 10 mg vitamin B6 may be enough. (Note: always take vitamin B6 with niacinamide.) In general, smaller amounts of vitamins taken throughout the day rather than one or two larger doses may be more successful.

- Taking DHEA tablets can be dangerous unless carefully monitored. If your DHEA levels are below normal, a low dose of micronized DHEA (5-10 mgs, twice daily) for a short period (one to two months) may be helpful. DHEA can increase estrogen, so avoid it if your estrogen levels are normal or above. DHEA can also slightly increase testosterone. Therefore, avoid DHEA if you have conditions associated with excess estrogen such as breast cancer or endometriosis, or conditions associated with excess testosterone such as prostate cancer. Long-term supplementation with DHEA can cause your adrenal glands to produce less of its own DHEA, making you dependent upon supplements.

Dietary Factors

For those with high cortisol, two major considerations include avoiding excess carbohydrates, and eating more frequently. Here are some other dietary guidelines that may help curb cortisol levels:

- Avoid sweets and meals high in refined carbohydrates (pasta, bread, etc.). Common symptoms indicating excess carbohydrate intake include stomach bloating, sleepiness or inability to focus mentally after a meal or snack, as described earlier.

- Consider eating a snack between your three main meals. Many people find eating every two to three hours helpful. Avoid sugars and refined starches, and fruit juice. Cheese, nuts, vegetables and half a meat or fish sandwich are some options.

- Avoid low-fat diets, as they can reduce certain hormone levels, such as testosterone. In addition, avoid low-cholesterol diets since cholesterol is a key component in the production of many hormones, including progesterone and testosterone.

- Always eat breakfast. Avoid refined cereals (nearly all cereals are refined and have added sugar). Whole eggs are part of an ideal breakfast.

- A variety of foods contain natural hormones, hormone precursors and substances that help regulate hormones. Foods most helpful to your hormone levels include soy, peanuts, licorice and yams. The most convenient foods include frozen green soy beans from your health-food store under the name SunRich. They're high in isoflavones, protein and relatively low in carbohydrates. Tofu is also a good source of soy, but don't eat frozen tofu desserts that are high in sugar, or processed soy products, which often contain monosodium glutamate (MSG), even though it's not listed as an ingredient. Examples of highly processed soy products which contain MSG are soy isolates, soy caseinates and hydrolyzed soy proteins.

- The use of licorice can help in some cases of adrenal-hormone imbalance. However, there are two different types of licorice extracts, and it's important to know your cortisol levels before taking any type of licorice. Regular licorice, such as the whole licorice-root extract commonly used, can raise cortisol. This is the type to use if your cortisol is too low, such as those under chronic stress or severely overtrained. It is contraindicated if your cortisol is already high (or even normal), and with conditions associated with high cortisol, such as high blood pressure. If your cortisol levels are too high, use de-glycyrrhized licorice instead of regular licorice, which can help lower cortisol.

- Reduce or eliminate caffeine which can raise cortisol levels.

Natural Hormone Creams

The best non-prescription hormone supplement for natural progesterone is Pro-Gest cream (Transitions for Health, Portland, Oregon). This is made from naturally occurring diosgenin found in the roots of wild yams. It is also useful when cortisol is high, and DHEA, estrogen and testosterone is low. It is difficult if not impossible to overdose yourself with natural progesterone.

Once in the body, natural progesterone produces small amounts of both estrogen and testosterone. As opposed to tablets, the cream helps moisten the skin, but most importantly, the natural hormone is not broken down in the liver as quickly as orally taken natural progesterone. Rub in about a half to a full teaspoon of cream after bathing on the soft skin of your arms, inner thighs or abdomen. Use for two to three weeks, then skip one to two weeks, or use as directed (an instruction pamphlet comes with the product explaining different uses for menopause, PMS, osteoporosis, etc.). Pro-Gest can be used by both women and men, as progesterone is converted to testosterone in males. Some notice positive effects within a week or two, with others requiring two to three months to see the difference. Liquid sublingual (under-the-tongue) progesterone is also useful and available without prescription.

John Lee, M.D., author of *Natural Progesterone* (BLL Publishing) suggests progesterone, rather than estrogen, for many common disorders, including PMS, menopausal symptoms, osteoporosis and others. It is important, however, that each person be treated as an individual, and that a complete assessment, including measurement of hormone levels, be performed before any therapy. Progesterone plays a vital role in the mineralization of bone. In the journal *Medical Hypothesis* (1991), Dr. Lee states, "The hypothesis that progesterone and not estrogen is the missing factor was tested in a clinical setting and was found to be extraordinarily effective in reversing osteoporosis."

When women are given hormone replacement therapy, the use of estrogen without progesterone (referred to as unopposed estrogen) can have significant and dangerous side effects. This can include uterine problems and breast cancer. Adding progesterone can prevent these problems. Unfortunately, synthetic progesterone (the most common ones being norethisterone and medroxyprogesterone acetate) also can have adverse effects, such as increased blood fats and poor sugar regulation, and can reduce the effectiveness of estrogen. Medical studies clearly show that the use of natural progesterone, which is identical to that made by the ovaries, has little or no side effects. Natural progesterone has been successfully used in Europe for more than 20 years.

Some women require additional estrogen for a variety of reasons: hot flashes, insomnia, bone loss, etc. For women who require both estrogen (more than can be converted from progesterone and DHEA) and progesterone, a natural cream called OstaDerm (Bezwecken, Beaverton, Oregon) is available. It's made from wild yam extracts, soybean, and licorice root as sources of natural phytoestrogens.

Other natural hormones are available, sometimes by prescription. For more information on doctors who prescribe natural hormones, call the Women's International Pharmacy (800-279-5708). The amount of natural hormone in many over-the-counter preparations is often very low — so be careful when using products you're not familiar with.

Evaluating your body's hormones can be done through symptom surveys and salivary hormone testing, and sometimes through other evaluations your doctor may request. In most cases of hormone imbalance, natural remedies are very effective. By improving hormone balance you'll not only be more healthy today, but in your later years as well. And, you'll be a healthier and more fit athlete who burns more body fat, has less injury and performs up to her potential.

18

Your Fat-Burning Profile

Most people think excess body "weight" and body "fat" are synonymous. The truth is that body fat, as a percentage of a person's weight, is influenced more by the body's water content than by any other single factor. For athletes, the obsession of "less is best" regarding body fat is another misconception. While athletic performance is influenced by and dependent upon the proportion and total amount of fat-free mass and fat mass, imbalances caused by forced reduction of body fat can produce serious problems. Both health and athletic performance can be reduced in individuals with too little body fat.

More than 25 percent of the adult population in the United States is overfat, with that number increasing all the time. Childhood obesity has also increased 20 percent during the last decade and is now prevalent in about 25 percent of U.S. children. Both groups, adults and children, have gotten fatter despite the population's overall reduction in dietary-fat consumption and increase in carbohydrate consumption. And athletes are not immune, either. While there are no accurate figures, I have seen great numbers of overfat endurance athletes, including professionals.

No "normal" body-fat levels should be established due to individual variations (i.e., physical and chemical body make-up). So I'm not going to give any percentages of body fat that athletes should strive to attain. Rather, improving your overall health and fitness should result in increased fat-burning. This will be evident in your clothes fitting more loosely, and you can also measure your waist-to-hip ratio as discussed in Chapter 14.

The traditional idea that weight control is easily accomplished by reducing kilocalories is oversimplified, as your metabolic state, i.e., how these kilocalories are burned, your level of carbohydrate tolerance, nutritional status and other issues are significant. More importantly, large amounts of weight loss, as seen in many fast weight-loss diets, is often short term, partly because the metabolic rate remains low, gradually bringing back the weight and body fat.

Assessment of Body Fat

It is best to use body-fat content as measured in the waist-to-hip ratio as a primary assessment tool, with scale weight as a secondary measurement, if used at all. As previously mentioned, I prefer stepping on the scale only before and after the Two-Week Test.

The waist-to-hip ratio may be the best single measurement that reflects metabolic function, especially in reference to burning off body fat. Measurements of body fat should not be taken daily or even weekly since fat loss takes place over a longer period of time. Frequent measurements may produce or maintain preoccupation as is often the case with individuals who are on a "diet" and weigh themselves on the scale once or twice a day. This can result in added stress, and stress itself can cause the body to store more fat.

The common devices and formulas used to measure body fat are very general, and neither precise nor comparable. For example, a study of bioelectrical impedance using 12 common formulas showed the formulas that performed well in one group gave poor results in another, and vice versa. Skinfold thickness, measured by calipers and using various formulas, may also vary in its assessment of fat content. For example, two identical skinfold thicknesses may have significantly different concentrations of fat cells. In addition, these external measurements of subcutaneous fat do not consider internal fat content. When calipers are compared to underwater weighing for body density, errors of 5 percent body fat — too large for accurate estimates — may be found. Even the use of more complex assessments, such as dual-energy X-ray absorptiometry, do not reveal precise measurements of body fat. Although more accurate, computerized analysis of magnetic resonance images also results in some variability, and are much less practical. In all, most of these methods underestimate body-fat content. The use of any device to obtain body-fat content should be considered only a very general measure, and you should understand that small changes are not relevant and may be due to error. A slight improvement in accuracy may be obtained if the same device is used in all evaluations, and by the same person.

As previously described, the use of respiratory quotient (RQ) can be a very accurate method to assess a person's metabolic changes. Although this test does not relate to body-fat content, it does determine the percentage of fat- and sugar-burning. As metabolism improves, and fat-burning increases, it is reflected in an improved RQ (the RQ lowers). This is almost always accompanied by body-fat reduction. And, people who burn more fat are protecting themselves against future increased fat storage. On the other hand, those with high body-fat content burn less fat for energy. This is reflected in a higher RQ not only in overfat patients, but in those at higher risk of future substantial body-fat gains, making high RQ a predictor of future fat gains.

The fact is, it may be difficult and too expensive for most athletes to continually go to a reputable lab for RQ analysis. Instead, perform the MAF test (see *Training for Endurance*) using the 180-Formula. This test parallels RQ levels most of the time. In other words, as you burn more body fat, your MAF test will improve (you get faster) along with your RQ.

Competitive Athletes and Weight Loss

Many athletes are overly conscious about their body fat. By eating too little, they risk not only reduced health but reduced performance as well. Studies show that restricting kilocalories as a means of losing body weight can result in diminished athletic performance. In addition, athletes who restrict energy intake to promote weight loss can also decrease bone density. The problem in some athletes is the increased mental/emotional pressure to attain low body weights — often inspired by years of looking at models in athletic magazines. As a result, athletes of all ages implement many unhealthy habits, including food restriction, especially fats, and in some cases dehydration (fluid restriction) or even bulimic behavior.

Clearly, more athletes than non-athletes are preoccupied with thoughts of eating and weight loss, have difficulty controlling body weight, abuse laxatives for weight control, and report disordered eating. Significant numbers of athletes use at least one method of weight control. There are a variety of over-the-counter weight-loss products used by athletes; laxatives and diuretics are the most common. One study found that an average of 29 percent of female athletes from several sports reported using weight-reducing products, with athletes from some sports showing very high levels, including those who play volleyball (71 percent). While most of these products do not reduce body fat, they can cause dehydration and potassium deficiency. Endurance athletes are not immune to this problem.

Diet and Nutrition

Although there are no special formulas for athletes with excess body fat, some key points should be reviewed here. Dietary assessment should be your initial evaluation. In their desire to restrict food, many athletes also restrict nutrient intake. This makes computerized dietary assessments — both initial and follow-up — very important. We must all be made aware of the importance of many nutrients necessary for balanced metabolism of carbohydrates, proteins and fats, as discussed in previous chapters. Many nutrients are important to increase the burning of body fat — especially the omega-6 and omega-3 balance. Chromium, vitamin B6, magnesium and others may be just as important. However, rather than consider a list of "fat-burning nutrients," realize that too-low levels of just about any nutrient can directly or indirectly impair the process of fat-burning. If you don't know your level of nutrient intake, you'll never know if certain nutrients are preventing you from burning more fat.

Among the most common problems associated with increased body fat is carbohydrate intolerance. This was discussed in detail in earlier chapters. Athletes eating a high-carbohydrate, low-fat diet usually utilize less fat for energy and rely more on sugar. A high-carbohydrate, low-fat diet may also worsen carbohydrate intolerance, setting you up for a vicious cycle of cravings for high-carbohydrate foods, more fat storage and eating more carbohydrates. Despite these and other clear indications that contraindicate low-fat, high-carbohydrate diets, they are still used for weight control by many athletes, and even by professionals. Unfortunately, this approach leads many to consume larger amounts of prepared low-fat foods, which are often made from high amounts of high-glycemic sugars that increase insulin prodution.

It may, therefore, be important for many athletes to begin the process of reducing body fat with a Two-Week Test. Recall also that food frequency is an important element in the dietary habits of those who want to control abnormal blood-sugar and insulin fluctuations. Spreading out the full day's food into many smaller meals rather than two or three large ones can significantly help produce more stable insulin and blood sugar, and can help burn more body fat. Many diet programs restrict meals and substitute high-carbohydrate drinks or other snacks, which are often a major metabolic stress for many athletes. It is important to emphasize that people should eat real food and real-food products throughout the day rather than rely on convenience items that are usually unhealthy, especially in relation to the balance of fats.

Other nutritional factors are often neglected in weight and fat loss:

- As discussed previously, fiber improves carbohydrate metabolism by decreasing the glycemic index of a meal. A general guide for the amount of fiber intake is at least 11g for each 1,000 kcal of food.

- Water is another important item, especially if protein intake is increased, which is often the case when total carbohydrate is lowered.

- It should also be noted that hot red peppers, which contain capsaicin, may have a positive effect in those who want to burn more body fat.

Training

For the majority of those who need to reduce body fat, the primary training focus is developing a good aerobic system. Many overfat athletes have excess anaerobic function and deficient aerobic function. Studies show that individuals with high body fat had increased proportions of anaerobic muscle fibers and decreased aerobic muscle fibers. The process of developing aerobic function should include regularly performing the MAF test, which will help measure progress and warn of impending plateau or regression of aerobic function. As noted above, improvements in the MAF test usually accompany body-fat loss.

Many athletes use exercise exclusively as a way of reducing body fat, and may be unsuccessful. One study that relied only on exercise showed that, of 31 overfat women, 20 lost substantial body fat, but 11 actually gained body fat, following six months of only aerobic training. They all showed similar improvements in VO_2 max, indicating they all benefited from their workouts. This study seems to indicate that without considering the whole person, including needs such as diet and nutrition, optimal success may not be attained.

It should be noted that athletes who have too little body fat can develop other problems, especially in women with amenorrhea, as discussed previously.

19

Shopping for Endurance

By now, it should be clear that proper nutrition is a must to supply the raw materials needed to help your body build more endurance. The importance of food preparation and having good meals and food available is also vital to accomplish this task. Even more important is how you shop — what to buy and what not to buy. What you put into your shopping cart is the same food that goes into your stomach once you get it home. Think of the shopping cart as your mouth, and be careful what you put into it.

There are generally two places you'll go for food. If you're fortunate enough to live in the country and have to go to one farm for eggs, and another for meat, in addition to other stores, you are lucky. Or perhaps there's a food co-op where healthy foods, along with organic items, can be bought for much less than retail. For the majority of athletes, some of your food will come from the large grocery chains, which have everything from apples to zucchini. Unfortunately, they also contain chemicals you probably would not even feed to your pet. A second location will probably be the modern "health-food" store — the misnomer being that all the food in these establishments is healthy. Regardless of where you shop, you'll have to think, plan ahead, and read labels before you buy.

Before venturing out to buy food, there are some things to consider:

- Know what you want to buy and make a list before you go. Don't be taken in by sales or ads (especially those little jingles still lingering in your head from last night's TV commercials).

- Don't shop if you're ready to drop. This means if your blood sugar is falling and you're getting hungry, don't go shopping. In this vulnerable condition, you're more likely to buy more junk food, especially sweets. Instead, eat first.

- If you're bringing your children, make sure they've eaten too. Stores stock many items at the eye level of youngsters to get their attention. The next thing you know, your children are asking (or telling) you to buy it. This is especially popular in the cereal isle. Popular cereals are loaded with sugar, bad fats and chemicals, and are among the worse foods to buy, especially for children.

- As you stroll through the store (I prefer a fast walk), look at the signs above the aisles so you know which aisle you're entering, rather than routinely traveling down them — the aisle less traveled means less temptation.

- Read the labels on items that have an ingredient list. This includes most products in grocery stores. If you're buying cheese and there's a whole paragraph of ingredients you can't pronounce, avoid it. Many people read the labels of foods they're buying for the first time, but don't realize that items they regularly buy contain ingredients they would not want to eat. Also, manufacturers sometimes change ingredients, so check those regular foods to make sure they're still OK.

- When the option exists, buy food grown in the United States rather than from other countries, where restrictions on pesticides and other pollutants may not be as high as the U.S. standards (not that the U.S. standards are good, they're just better than many other places). European foods are the exception, as their standards are generally much higher than in the United States.

- Generally restrict or avoid foods not normally grown in your geographical region. For example, if you live in the north, eat apples more often than oranges. If you live in New York, potatoes from the East Coast are preferred over those grown in Idaho.

- Never, ever taste any of the free samples they're trying to give out in the grocery-store aisles. This is a popular trend in many areas of the country. These items are almost without exception highly processed and full of chemicals and sugar.

- In general, there are usually healthier, or more natural versions of your favorite foods. For example, whole-rye crackers instead of saltines, fresh ginger instead of the packaged version which contains sugar and coloring, canola mayonnaise instead of the mayo with hydrogenated fat.

- Avoid buying produce, fruits, meats or cheese that has been cut or chopped up. Try to buy the whole item. For example, buy whole heads of leaf lettuce rather than bags that have been pre-chopped. Chopping causes vitamins to be lost and more rapid deterioration of the food. In addition, stores often do this with the stray leaves that are left after the better-looking heads are displayed.

- To remove some of the pesticide from your fruits and vegetables, wash them whole in warm water with a very mild "safe" soap solution (Dr. Bronner's unscented soap is a good one), and rinse with plain water. This will also remove the waxy stuff groceries spray on peppers, cucumbers, apples, and many other foods to make them shiny.

Grocery Stores

At your local grocery, you'll find everything. But that doesn't mean you should buy it. There may be certain items you'll need at these outlets, depending on how aware you are of foods, chemicals and the environment. For example, the use of laundry soap can be almost eliminated by using the small washing-machine discs, which work amazingly well and are now becoming popular. Or, if you believe that plain synthetic vitamin C (which is just ascorbic acid) sold in most groceries today, is better than a vitamin C complex (which includes bioflavonoids and other substances), so be it.

What you buy and don't buy here also depends on your discipline, and belief in real food. If you really believe Wonder bread builds strong bodies 12 ways (the Federal Trade Commission finally made the company stop advertising that claim) and bologna is really good for you, so be it.

A trip to the grocery may get you some standard paper products — towels, toilet paper, napkins, perhaps some coffee filters (the brown ones are without bleach), and a number of other products that are just made from food — sauerkraut, olives, mustard, rye crackers, extra-virgin olive oil, etc. Check the labels on these foods too, just to be sure there are no unwanted ingredients.

In addition, a variety of fresh fruits and vegetables may come from the grocery store. The question is, are you willing to buy organic food if you have to travel farther or pay a little more? My recommendation is a resounding "yes!" Even considering that perhaps, just perhaps, they're not any better than the regular stuff, but contain less chemicals, I still think it's worth it.

You probably can't buy all your fruits and vegetables this way, but many seasonal ones are available in many areas. This leaves produce like garlic, onions, ginger root, and a variety of other fresh vegetables, and perhaps most fruits, to buy at your local grocery. Look for seasonal ones, and don't buy "green" food — the unripe products that should change color as they ripen, but which stores would rather sell you green. These include green peppers (they turn red, yellow, orange or purple), tomatoes (of course they're red, sometimes yellow), bananas (of course, yellow) and even limes (which turn yellow). These ripened foods not only taste better but have more nutrients.

Try to buy all your vegetables fresh, with only an occasional frozen one as a second choice. With these two options almost always available, there's no reason to eat canned vegetables. An exception is canned vine-ripened tomatoes, which contain little or no preservatives or other chemicals.

"Health-Food" Stores

An equal amount of time and money may be spent in specialty shops, most often the common "health-food" store. These contain items that the large chain grocer is only beginning to stock, as well as many items which can only be found in health-food stores. For example, real, 100-percent whole-grain breads are difficult to find anywhere else. I like the sprouted multigrain types, usually frozen for longer shelf life.

A more common question previously asked has to be answered again — do you want to pay more for organic products? Organic brown rice, for example, may cost a little more; but I prefer that over the regular. Items which you don't use large amounts of every day, such as butter or sour cream, are best bought organic in hopes of not having the chemicals and hormones which may be found in regular brand-name products.

Especially if you have children, the more items bought in a health-food store, organic co-op, or which are local or home-grown without chemicals, the fewer harmful substances children will get into their sensitive, growing bodies. Don't wait for a medical study to reveal that chemical X causes disease Y to stop using something, when the connection has been suspected for years. Such is the case with many chemicals and otherwise adulterated foods and food ingredients.

Some people ask, how do you know if these foods are really organic? Today, there are government standards, so it's not nearly the risk it once was. The real answer, however, is that I'd rather gamble. I think it's better than to risk eating something I know contains unhealthy chemicals.

Food from the Farm

Many people, most of them unknowingly, have foods available that can be bought on a local farm, or in a market supplied by such a farm. More and more, farms are growing food that do not have, or contain safer or minimal amounts of chemicals you're trying to avoid. For example, my beef is from a farm that does not use chemicals and hormones, and allows the cows to roam the fields. At $1.60 a pound (for a quarter, half or whole cow), it's a great bargain. Having a large freezer is necessary in this endeavor. It will pay for itself quickly.

The same is true for chicken. If you knew how chickens were raised and the chemicals they contained, you'd never buy one again in a regular store. So-called free-range chickens are becoming popular, and usually cost more, although not necessarily if you find a good farm. Sometimes, however, these chickens may not be as free-range as you think.

The same is true with other foods, especially eggs. It's worth buying higher-quality, organic or free-range eggs. Nothing is more sensitive to its environment than a laying hen. If the feed is good, they'll lay good eggs. If it's cheap and full of chemicals, that's just what you'll get in your eggs. In Greece and other areas in Europe, eggs high in omega-3 fats are commonly available, due to the feed containing the same. This is starting to become popular in the United States and many chain grocery stores already are stocking this type of eggs.

Of course, nothing beats growing your own organic food. This can be the traditional summer garden, easy-to-grow spring and fall crops, and even winter crops, whether you're in northern or southern climates. For example, a cold frame in the snow belt will easily grow enough lettuce for a family of four. And, by freezing or canning your garden foods, you'll have a higher-quality product than the fresh version available in most stores during the winter.

If you have a little more room, chickens are easy and cheap to maintain. They'll eat the leftovers from your kitchen, bugs in the garden, even their own egg shells. A good hen will average about one egg per day, less in northern winters.

Going shopping should be a very high priority, since that's the primary source of your meals and snacks. More and more, online shopping (via the Internet) will be popular, even for fresh foods. But until then, before venturing out, carefully plan ahead, don't shop hungry, read labels and spend the extra money on important food items that add nutrition and restrict chemicals. Skimp on paper products, cosmetics, toiletries and other truly less-important items.

20

Endurance Foods: Best and Worst

This chapter reviews foods you want to regularly include in your diet if your goal is improved endurance, and overall better health. It also lists those foods that you want to avoid — as much as possible — to avoid impairing your endurance and health. Most of the issues listed here have been discussed in previous chapters.

Best Foods

- Carbohydrates: brown rice, beans, fresh fruits (eat less of the high-glycemic fruits such as grapes, bananas and oranges) and berries.
- Proteins: whole eggs, beef, fish and unprocessed soy.
- Fats: extra-virgin olive, avocado and flaxseed oil.
- All fresh vegetables (except potatoes and corn). Eat a variety as the season permits, especially onions and garlic.
- Fresh ginger.
- Nuts: especially almonds, cashews, macadamias and walnuts.
- Almond butter.
- Water — free of chlorine and fluoride.

Note: *Eat some raw food at each meal. If possible buy as much organic food or grow some of your own. Buy organic or otherwise chemical- and hormone-free eggs and meats.*

Best Regular Supplements

- Those containing whole foods or isolated nutrients rather than synthetics.
  - — Certified toxin-free EPA fish oil, in capsules or perles to prevent oxidation, or flaxseed oil.
  - — Raw sesame-seed oil in capsules or perles.
  - — Chromium in whole-food forms.

Worst Foods

The worst foods to eat include those that your body cannot tolerate, such as foods that may trigger allergies, cause intestinal stress or those to which you have an aversion. If you have an aversion to all the "Best Foods," you have a problem.

- **Carbohydrates:** If you are allergic to gliadin-containing foods (gliadin is a common allergen) these should be avoided. This can be indicated by a blood test, salivary test or food trial. Gliadin-containing foods include wheat, oats, rye, barley, wheat germ and most other grains, but not most legumes. Most grains also contain high amounts of phytic acid, which impair absorption of calcium, magnesium, iron and zinc.
- **High-glycemic carbohydrates:** These include all processed flour (most bread, pasta, rolls, bagels, cereals), sugar and sugar-containing foods (sweets, desserts, etc. — read the labels), potatoes, corn, high-sugar bars and sports drinks, and dried fruit, including raisins. However, during your workout or when racing, high-glycemic foods and drinks can be of value.
- **Protein:** Processed proteins, included hydrolyzed protein and those labeled as isolates or caseinates, and ground meat (unless ground right before eating) should be avoided.
- **Fats:** Overheated oils (fried foods), margarine and other fats that have been hydrogenated or partially hydrogenated, excess saturated fat, and excess omega-6 fat (oils of peanut, safflower, corn, soy, and most oils in common use).
- **Fruits and vegetables:** Avoid unripe fruits and vegetables. Green peppers turn red, yellow or purple when ripe. Also ripe bananas

should be yellow and ripe tomatoes should be red. Even limes should turn yellow when ripe.

Worst Supplements

- Synthetic vitamin products, especially those used to fortified foods.
- Vitamin D, vitamin D-containing supplements and food fortified with vitamin D. Athletes already get more than enough from the sun.
- Use of antacids for calcium.
- Dolomite as a calcium supplement.
- High-dose vitamin and mineral products, unless specifically prescribed by a professional.

Foods to Limit

- Fluoridated water.
- Overcooked food.
- Milk and milk-containing products (read the labels).
- Thiaminase-containing foods; these include *raw* versions of the following: red chicory, Brussels sprouts, red cabbage, clams, oysters, squids and other mollusks, herring and smelt.

21

Dairy: Milking Your Health

When the American Academy of Pediatrics suggested kids with certain problems avoid drinking cow's milk, and to not feed it to infants under one year of age, the advertisements for milk suddenly increased dramatically across the United States. Unfortunately, most people still hear the milk ads much louder than any professional recommendations. Milk consumption is up, and so are the problems created by it.

Even adults who drink milk should think twice about it. In many people, milk can cause various types of gastrointestinal stress, skin problems and lowered immunity, making you more susceptible to infections and allergies. Many experts agree that humans should not make cow's milk part of their diet. The old axiom is "cow's milk is for calves, human milk is for humans."

The problems associated with cow's milk start early. Milk may be a common cause of anemia in infants, and its consumption later in childhood may contribute to the development of type I diabetes. Milk allergies are very common in children and cause sinus problems, diarrhea, constipation and fatigue. Milk is a leading cause of chronic ear infections which plague up to 40 percent of children under the age of 6. Milk allergies are also linked to behavioral problems in children, and sometimes to childhood asthma. Milk allergies are equally common in adults and produce similar symptoms.

Milk Hormones and Cancer

The Food and Drug Administration approves the use of bovine growth hormone in cows. This increases milk production by up to 25 percent. This chemical hormone is associated with the growth of cancer cells, specifically breast cancer in women. Dr. J. L. Outwater of the Physicians Committee For Responsible Medicine in Washington, D.C., states, "Dairy products contain both hormones and growth factors, in addition to fat and various chemical contaminants, that have been implicated in the proliferation of human breast-cancer cells." In addition, these same chemicals are associated with increased prostate cancer in men, and cancers of the intestinal tract. Growth hormone stimulates the production of high levels of insulin-like growth factor-1 (IGF-1), which is the real culprit. The more growth hormone given to the cow, the more IGF-1 in its milk. Worse is that infants can absorb more of this substance than can adults. And, pasteurization further increases IGF-1. When drinking a 12-oz. glass of milk, you double the amount of IGF-1 in your body.

High levels of growth hormone can also increase infections of the cow's udders, which results in the use of more antibiotics and therefore higher traces of these drugs, as well as pus and bacteria from infected udders, found in their milk.

Udder infection is measured by estimating the number of somatic cells (pus cells) found in milk. In most cases, dairy farmers are allowed up to 50,000 live bacteria cells per gram of milk — this is considered safe and ready to go to market. That's millions of bacteria in each gulp. Some milk not allowed on the market due to high bacteria counts is made into powdered or dry milk and is allowed to be sold as such.

The proteins in cow's milk are much different and more difficult for the human intestinal tract to digest and for the immune system to tolerate. For example, cow's milk is about 80 percent casein and 20 percent whey; human milk is just the opposite, at 20 percent casein and 80 percent whey. It's the casein that causes the allergic and hypersensitivity reactions in both infants and adults. Even Dr. Benjamin Spock, M.D., America's greatest pediatrician, described casein as the primary cause of mucus, congestion and childhood earaches.

Milk's lactose is another potential problem as some people have lactose intolerance, which will be described later.

Goat's Milk

Human milk is very unique. The milk that comes closest to our own is goat milk (actually rat milk is closer to human milk, but I don't suggest trying to find any). If you still want to consume milk, there are a number of benefits to drinking goat's milk over cow's milk:

- Higher levels of B vitamins and better balance of minerals (the overall nutrient content is much closer to that of human milk).
- The mild laxative action of goat's milk aids the digestive process.
- The high buffering quality of goat's milk enhances its value for sufferers of peptic ulcers and other stomach problems.

Drinking goat's milk will benefit those who are unable to digest the high casein (protein) content in cow's milk. However, it will not necessarily help those who have lactose intolerance as goat's milk also contains lactose, though in lower quantities. As mentioned previously, the American Academy of Pediatrics suggests not using cow's milk or goat's milk for babies under 1 year of age.

The fat globules in goat's milk are smaller, finer, and more evenly distributed throughout the milk. As a result, goat's milk is naturally homogenized, and does not have to be treated like cow's milk, which is homogenized by adding certain chemicals to prevent the fat globules from floating to the top.

As with infant diets, the value of goat's milk for adults lies in the direct replacement of cow's milk, and thus the reduction in allergenic reaction to the cow's milk protein. And, goat's milk has a much lower level of lactose (a high-glycemic sugar), a consideration important for those who are carbohydrate intolerant, including diabetics.

As noted, goat's milk is higher in whey protein, as opposed to the highly allergenic casein protein of cow's milk. Whey proteins can have a positive influence on your immune system, and are a very high-quality protein. Avoid whey that is labeled isolated or hydrolyzed.

Milk Allergy and Lactose Intolerance

There are two separate issues when it comes to adverse reactions from milk and other dairy products. Milk allergy is relatively common, and lactose intolerance is much less common. However, there are still many people who do not effectively digest lactose, with the result being intestinal distress and sometimes inflammation.

A milk allergy is a true allergic reaction by the body's immune system to casein, the milk's protein (sometimes it's another protein, lactoglobulin, that triggers the allergy). Most of the time, symptoms are immediate and typically include swelling, itching, hives, abdominal cramping, breathing difficulty and diarrhea. Sometimes, chronic constipation is the result. In a severe reaction, hypotension or shock can result.

Many babies are born with allergies to cow's milk. They may not grow out of their allergies and can be affected throughout their life, sometimes without knowing why. As a result, many adults with hard-to-diagnose skin disorders, respiratory problems, gastric upsets, asthma, and even headaches, may have milk allergies. Many of these people can tolerate goat's milk.

Many milk allergies are sometimes referred to as hypersensitivities. Regardless of the name, these problems in adults, typically occurring as gastrointestinal reactions, may be more common than previously thought. These individuals may also have less problems when they take lactobacillus acidophilus, bulgaricus or other cultures (as found in yogurt), or from supplements such as L-Glutamine Plus (Nutri West).

Lactose intolerance is not an allergy. In this condition the digestive system does not produce enough of an enzyme called lactase, which breaks down the complex lactose sugar into simpler sugars. The lactose sugar ferments in the small intestine, producing gas, bloating, cramps and diarrhea. Adult humans, like all full-grown animals, often lose their ability to produce lactase enzyme and therefore can not adequately digest lactose. Human adult-onset lactase decline is normal in the intestine in the majority of the world's population. The problem is even more common in a majority of people of African, Asian, Hispanic and Native-American descent.

It may be best to distinguish between those with true lactose intolerance, and those who poorly digest lactose. The latter group is much more prevalent. A study by A. Carroccio, et al. (*Journal of the American College of Nutrition*, 1998) conducted at a rural clinic in Italy, showed that 32.2 percent of test subjects digested lactose poorly, while 4 percent were clearly lactose intolerant.

Foods to predominantly avoid if you have any adverse reactions to lactose include milk, skim milk and powdered milk. Heavy cream and butter, for example, contain no (or no significant amount) of lactose. The amount of lactose in cheese and yogurt depends upon how it was processed and the source of milk. Most people with lactose intolerance can usually tolerate lactose in small doses. Professionals can diagnose this problem with a breath hydrogen level test. You can usually self-assess this problem by avoiding foods containing lactose for a couple of weeks to see if you feel better. Then add a moderate amount to your next few meals and observe for a return of symptoms.

Most cheese does not contain lactose. The exceptions include whey cheeses which contain some lactose. Most commercial yogurt still contains moderate amounts of lactose because it has not been fermented very long. If you want yogurt without lactose, make your own by fermenting it for 24 hours rather than the usual 8-12. This provides the bacteria in the yogurt ample time to digest all the lactose.

Of interest for some people with lactose intolerance or for those who poorly digest lactose is the association of these problems with irritable bowel syndrome, premenstrual syndrome and mental depression.

LACTOSE-CONTAINING DAIRY	LACTOSE-FREE DAIRY
• Milk (liquid, dry, milk solids)	• Home-made yogurt (24-hour process)
• Sour cream (read labels)	• Cheese (partial list):
• Some cheeses	– Blue
– Cottage	– Cheddar
– Cream	– Edam
– Mozzarella	– Gouda
– Ricotta	– Havarti
– Feta	– Monterey Jack
– Most processed cheese	– Muenster
• Ice cream	• Dry-curd (uncreamed) cottage cheese (also called baker's, farmer's or hoop cheese)
• Ice milk	
• Half and half	
• Commercial yogurt	

Calcium Foods

If you decide to reduce your dairy intake, you must assure yourself that your diet contains enough calcium from other sources. This is not difficult to do if your diet is well rounded. The fact that milk and other dairy contains calcium does not necessarily mean you'll absorb it. In fact, calcium from kale, for example, is absorbed significantly better than milk. Oxalate-rich vegetables, such as spinach, have a lower rate of calcium absorption. Compared to a glass of 2 percent milk (calcium content of 297 mg) the following single servings contain high amounts of calcium:

Almonds	**100 mg**
Collards	**125 mg**
Green beans	**100 mg**
Rainbow trout	**100 mg**
Salmon	**225 mg**
Sardines	**115 mg**
Seaweed	**140 mg**
Soybeans	**175 mg**
Spinach	**135 mg**

If you ate one of each of the above items during the course of the day, you'd get 1,215 mg of calcium, not including the calcium in other foods. If you eat several servings of vegetables, you're likely to get a large amount of calcium. Or, combining certain foods can really boost calcium intake: a three-egg vegetable omelet, for example, can provide more calcium than a glass of milk.

Or, try this: Put about a dozen's worth of clean eggshells from your morning breakfasts into a small bottle of vinegar. This will both "sweeten" the vinegar and provide a tremendous amount of calcium from the eggshells. Use it on salad as part of an oil-and-vinegar dressing. You'll get a lot more calcium this way than you ever will from antacids.

22

Snacks for Endurance

As previously discussed, snacks, or mini-meals, can help reduce adrenal-gland stress, control excess insulin production and stabilize blood sugar. It's also helpful for weight loss and burning body fat. It's important to keep a variety of healthy snack foods on hand at all times, so make plans for your snacking habits when you shop. Here are some snacking ideas:

- Use leftovers for your next snack. For example, prepare or buy more for lunch and save some of it for your snack. This can also work with other meals. For example, if you're having quiche for breakfast, save a piece for a snack. Save part of your large dinner for the next day's snack.

- Nuts. Preferably raw almonds or cashews.

- Almond butter, spread on whole-grain crackers, or fresh apple or pear slices, is delicious.

- A quick smoothie makes a great snack: Plain yogurt and fresh fruit, blended, are all you need. As an option, try adding nut butter, an egg yolk or two (no whites, as they contain an enzyme that shouldn't be eaten raw) or a small amount of vanilla or almond extract.

- Cheese can be part of a great snack with fruit or nuts, or eaten by itself.

- Soup. Make a big pot and freeze in small amounts. That way, you'll always have some available for a snack. Hearty vegetable soups with meat, fish, and smaller amounts of beans or rice, are great snacks or meals.
- Snacks should be of the same proportion as your meals. If eating meals that are lower in carbohydrates, and moderate in protein and fat makes you feel the best, your snacks should be similar.
- Use whole-food, prepackaged snacks such as Phil's Bars. They store well, travel well and are convenient.
- A piece of fruit. Fruit is easy to travel with, store and eat. Even a container of berries makes an easy snack.
- Hard-boiled eggs. They are easy to store and travel well. Try boiling, peeling and salting them ahead of time. You can boil enough eggs for a few days worth of snacks. An egg or two with a raw vegetable such as a carrot or stick of celery makes a great snack.
- Made-ahead tuna or egg salad is also a good option.

Snacks can help maintain and improve the efficiency of your metabolism, which will in turn improve your endurance.

23

Making Good Bad Choices

Eating on the run is something most of us do at some time. Unfortunately too many people do this more often than eating a peaceful, healthy meal. I believe it's just a matter of setting priorities, something essential if you wish to consume the right foods for a balanced diet.

Nonetheless, there will be a time when eating on the run is the only option. Many times, unexpected delays or changes in schedules force you to make this unsavory decision. But it should be done only when absolutely necessary, when the other option is not eating at all — an option many should avoid. I usually pack food when traveling. But that's not always possible, and on longer trips I sometimes run out of food. Here are some dos and don'ts for those days.

- Avoid eating on the run. I know that's what this section is about, but if you plan to avoid it, you may find you do it less.

- Plan ahead. If you think about lunch the evening before you find yourself hungry and driving past "fast-food alley" you'll know where you're going to get a meal — from a small cooler of food you've packed.

- For a day on the road, or your regular commute, bring food in your car, on the train or plane or wherever you're going. Although not as nice, pretend you're going on a picnic. Don't worry about what others are thinking or smelling — they only wish they were as organized as you are. Under no circumstances should this be done in place of sitting down to a meal just to save time. Wake up a few minutes earlier, or plan ahead so you don't have to eat this way.

- If you're going to a familiar location, know where the good stores or restaurants are located. Keep a log of these locations if you plan on visiting the same place again. Get a take-out menu or a book of matches from the restaurant and keep it in your car or at home for easy reference.
- Avoid eating foods you don't like, or items that don't agree with you. Many people tend to eat at places they are familiar with rather than places that are good. Remember which restaurant chains are OK and which are not.
- When choosing hotels, stay at the ones that have at least a coffee pot and refrigerator. (Ask when making your reservation.) Bring your own coffee or tea, as well as your own food.
- If you're staying at a hotel, especially for more than a day or two, use the refrigerator much like you do at home. Some hotel refrigerators are filled with liquor and junk food — remove it and neatly put it alongside the refrigerator (so the hotel doesn't charge you for it). Now there's room for your real food.
- Bring good food from home. Kept in the freezer the previous day or two, most food is safe during travel, especially if it's in an insulated bag. Just make sure it doesn't stay frozen so long you can't eat it.
- When eating in the restaurant, order more than you'll eat and bring leftovers back to your room for a later snack or meal.
- If you're going to be in a hotel more than a few days, go food shopping for things you can eat in your room. If that's not easy to do, save food at each meal ordered out for later use.
- Have some basic utensils in your suitcase at all times: plastic forks, knives and spoons. Or, order room service the first day and save (and rinse) the utensils.

- Travel with plates and bowls as needed.
- Always carry a pocketknife.
- A coffee pot is not only useful for coffee and tea, but for heating food.
- Rather than submitting to just eating junk food, be selective (see "When Eating Junk Food" below).
- Carry water with you. If you're on the road for more than a day or two, bring a small portable water filter to replenish your water bottle. If you're stuck somewhere without water, most fast-food places, delis and restaurants will give (or sell) you a "to go" cup with water.

When Eating Junk Food

When your choices are limited to junk food, it's best to pick the least deadly substances. Here's a list of the best junk food if and when you have to make a choice:

- Pizza (thin crust). If you can get it with vegetables, that's even better. Stay away from the popular pizza chains and try to find the local family pizzeria, which tend to use more real-food ingredients.
- It's usually easy to find a deli. Most large grocery chains have them now. Most people don't think of a deli as "fast food," but much of the food in there is highly processed — just read the labels on the meats. If you can find a large health-food store chain with a deli, the food is usually of a higher quality, less processed and contains less chemicals. Some of these delis even have sushi to go.
- Stick with the meats that are closer to real — turkey breast, roast beef or ham — rather than the highly processed choices like olive loaf, hot dogs or meat patties. Still, roast beef is usually not just roast beef — it often contains sugar and chemicals to add taste and preserve the meat. Ask to see the list of ingredients.

- Consider an egg sandwich from a deli (or diner), maybe with ham if you're really hungry. Sometimes they only make egg sandwiches in the morning, but many will prepare them anytime.

- Many delis also serve hot food — make sure it's not fried (eggplant, chicken, veal parmigiana).

- If you're not intolerant to dairy, eat some real cheese as a snack or a sandwich. Avoid the "American" cheese and cheese spreads.

- Dying for some chocolate? Find the real thing. A small bar of real chocolate, one which contains few ingredients, is usually not terribly high in sugar and is milk-free. A small piece will usually satisfy that junk-food craving.

- Avoid the fried foods. If you have to make the unfortunate choice of a fried fish fillet and a grilled hamburger, choose the latter. Bad fats can stay in your body for months, continually affecting your metabolism.

For many people, going hungry can be a major stress on the body. When the choices are limited to bad ones, make the best one.

24

The 10 Commandments of Cooking

Proper meal preparation is vital to good health and central to eating for endurance. How you prepare the food you'll eat and the foods you choose as ingredients for creating meals can significantly impact your body chemistry and the mechanisms that control digestion and absorption, energy production, hormone balance and other key factors.

Below are the "10 commandments" of cooking, things to do and not to do in the process of preparing your meals.

1. Never use hydrogenated or partially hydrogenated fats such as margarine or shortening, or oils labeled as having these substances. Use only unsalted "sweet" butter (the highest-quality butter fat), or extra-virgin olive oil.

2. Never overheat oil, especially when sautéing your food in oil. Instead, steam your vegetables, bake or broil your meats and fish, or pan-fry using the fat naturally found in the food (for example, a pan-fried steak). Avoid using oils for baking — use butter instead. If an oil is necessary in sautéing or baking, use extra-virgin olive oil.

3. When steaming or boiling, never use more water than necessary. Steaming is preferable to boiling. Use what

water does remain after cooking vegetables in soups or for other cooking, or drink with sea salt as a tea. Many vitamins and minerals are lost in the water in which foods are cooked.

4. Never overcook your food. Soft-cooked eggs are preferred over hard-boiled or scrambled; rare meat is better than medium or well-done. Lightly steam vegetables rather than boiling or frying them. This is especially true for fish, which tastes "fishy" even when slightly overcooked.

5. Use whole foods as ingredients instead of processed ones. For example, use whole oats for oatmeal instead of the quick-cook type which are processed, or brown rice instead of "minute rice." The less your food is adulterated by the manufacturer or grocer, the better. In general, make meals from real food rather than buying processed, precooked or ready-to-eat items.

6. Avoid ground meat unless it has been freshly ground the same day. The same is true of foods made with ground meats (hot dogs, sausages, meat patties, etc.). Make it fresh or avoid it.

7. Use fresh foods first, frozen when fresh is not available, and canned as a last resort.

8. Include some raw food at each meal prepared. Avocado, soft-cooked egg yolk, tomato or other garnish, etc.

9. Use only sea salt when salting. Ideally use coarse salt and grind as needed.

10. Presentation is important. Make meals not only healthy and tasty, but also attractive to the eye. For example, a variety of colors is not only more healthy but pleasing to the eye (this actually will help you digest better).

Abiding by these 10 commandments when cooking will help you make healthy meals when eating for endurance.

25

Eating for Kids

Babies are born endurance athletes. As adults we can influence them in a positive, healthy way from the time they are born (actually even before). Or we can allow others to have a negative, unhealthy influence. These bad influences come in the form of tradition, marketing and advertising, and convenience. In addition to treating many children as patients in practice, I'm also a father and grandfather, so my experience is real.

During my years of practice, I had many children as patients, and the most important feature was that kids respond very well (better than adults) to natural remedies. And, maintaining good health is also relatively easy. My experience included my own three children, and now, my grandchildren. However, children are also just as easily harmed by poor diets and nutritional deficiencies. Most frightening is how vulnerable they are to advertisements and media hype. So it's more important to counter that propaganda with proper habits and healthy, rational discussions, beginning at a very early age.

Perhaps more alarming is that most often, functional health problems are not initially very obvious. Most pediatricians are experts at ruling out serious conditions, but may fail to notice functional imbalances. Kids can have nutritional and exercise imbalances without accompanying signs and symptoms for a long time. Only after a period of time will earlier imbalances begin to cause more obvious trouble. This comes in the form of increased body fat, allergies, cavities (yes, they're preventable with proper nutrition), or often the so-called "growing pains," which are problems unexplained by traditional medicine. But these problems are usually functional in nature and are treatable. Also included are behavioral problems, learning difficulties and other common issues parents face.

The best treatment for kids is a good lifestyle, proper diet and good nutrition. Many parents have asked me if it's still possible to get the benefits from these three factors even if they didn't start out right. Of course it is. But you can't start too soon.

Here are some general healthy-living rules for children:

- Breastfeeding is more than just best. As the baby's first food, it's the only real option for healthy mothers.
- Do not feed babies anything other than mother's milk for at least six months (not even water).
- Slowly introducing new foods to infants may be best in this order: vegetables, fruits, eggs, meats, grains and dairy. Avoid milk, except goat's milk. Never give your child fruit juice.
- Allow kids to eat as much or as little as they want, as long as it's real food. They intuitively know what they need.
- Encourage raw vegetables and fruits at each meal. For children who are eating solid foods, blend raw fruits and vegetables in a Cuisinart.
- Always have enough healthy food options — especially a variety of fresh foods.
- Buy organic foods as much as possible. Pesticides, hormones and other chemicals in our food supply can be more harmful to the growing bodies of youngsters than to those of adults. It's worth spending a few pennies more per meal for the higher-quality foods.
- Introduce water early (after 6 months) and encourage its use. Avoid chlorinated and fluorinated water. Water should be the main liquid.
- Strictly avoid all soda, cereals, bad oils (hydrogenated, palm and palm kernel, and fried foods to name some) and sugar-laced foods.

- The 1995 Dietary Guidelines for Americans (USDA) does not recommend restricting fat intake for children under age 2 (and by age 5 the diet should be no more than 30 percent fat). Restricting fat can result in reduced calcium, iron and protein intakes, and can impair growth. The Canadian Pediatric Society recommends kids maintain an higher than 30 percent fat diet until age 18.

Kids eating a high-carbohydrate diet may be at risk for increased triglycerides and lower HDL cholesterol (a higher risk for heart disease) later in life (sometimes not so late). Specifically, use sweets sparingly. When you do use them, avoid those with chemicals and highly processed foods. Poor carbohydrate metabolism may be indicated if your child has one or more of the following signs or symptoms:

- ❑ Low birth weight (less than 5.5 pounds)
- ❑ Taller than average for age
- ❑ Increased weight or body fat
- ❑ Sleep problems
- ❑ Mother: increased stress during pregnancy
- ❑ Increased aggression or anger
- ❑ Hyperactive
- ❑ Attention Deficit Disorder (ADD)
- ❑ Overeating sweets or carbohydrates upsets
- ❑ Athletic activity low

In addition, activity is vital to good health. Unfortunately, today's children are generally very inactive, often due to excess television viewing. Encourage daily activity. Your child's future health is in your hands; so is the health of their children, and their children's children.

Appendix A: Glycemic Index

Some common foods and food groups and their average glycemic-index listing, using white bread as the standard (GI = 100) (adapted from Poster-Powell and Miller 1995).

FOOD	GI
Sugars	
Honey	104
Sucrose	92
Maltose	150
Glucose	138
Fructose	32
White bread	100
Whole-grain bread	52-73
Cakes and muffins	70-102
Soft drinks	97
Bagel	103
Rolls	90-106
Cereals	
All-Bran	45-75
Cheerios	106
Corn Flakes	110-130
Cream of Wheat	94-105
Crispix	124
Grapenuts	96
Nutri-grain	94
Total	109
Oatmeal	77
One-Minute Oats	94
Puffed Wheat	96-114
Rice Crispies	117
Shredded Wheat	83-118
Special K	77
White rice	71-83
Instant rice	128
Brown rice	79
Pasta (average)	68
Fresh fruits	
Apple	52
Apricots	44
Bananas	76
Cherries	32
Grapefruit	36
Grapes	62
Orange	62
Peach	40
Pear	51
Pineapple	94
Plums	34
Raisins	91
Watermelon	103
Dairy foods	
Full fat milk	39
Skim milk	46
Yogurt with fruit	47
Legumes	
Baked beans	69
Chick peas	47
Kidney beans	42
Green beans	42
Pinto beans	59
Soy beans	25
Lentils	41
Peanuts	21
Vegetables	
Beets (root)	91
Carrots	101
White, baked potatoes	121
Boiled potatoes	80
New potatoes	81
French-fried potatoes	107
Sweet corn	78
Peas	68
Yams	73

Appendix B: References

Adams P, et al. (1996). Arachidonic acid to eicosapentaenoic acid ratio in blood correlates positively with clinical symptoms of depression. Lipids; 31 Suppl:S157-S161.

Aitken JC, Thompson J (1989). The effects of dietary manipulation upon the respiratory exchange ratio as a predictor of maximum oxygen uptake during fixed term maximal incremental exercise in man. Eur J Appl Physiol 58: 722-727.

Alessio HM, et al. (1997). Exercise-induced oxidative stress before and after vitamin C supplementation. Int J Sport Nutr 7(1): 1-9.

Arena B, et al. (1995). Reproductive hormones and menstrual changes with exercise in female athletes. Sports Med 19(4): 278-287.

Armstrong LE, et al. (1994). Urinary indices of hydration status. Int J Sport Nutr 4(3): 265-279.

Balon R, et al. (1989). Family history of anxiety disorders in control subjects with lactate-induced panic attacks. Am J Psychiatry 146: 1304-1306.

Benson JE, et al. (1996). Nutritional aspects of amenorrhea in the female athlete triad. Int J Sport Nutr 6(2): 134-145.

Bergman EA, et al. (1990). Effects of dietary caffeine on renal handling of minerals in adult women. Life Sci 47(6): 557-564.

Bergstrom J, et al. (1990). Effect of a test meal, without and with protein, on muscle and plasma free amino acids. Clin Sci (Colch) 79(4): 31-337.

Bird SR, Hay S (1987). Pre-exercise food and heart rate during submaximal exercise. Br J Sports Med 21(1): 27-28.

Bjorntorp, P (1991). Importance of fat as a support nutrient for energy: metabolism of athletes. J Sports Sci 9: 71-76.

Bosch AN, et al. (1994). Influence of carbohydrate ingestion on fuel substrate turnover and oxidation during prolonged exercise. J Appl Physiol 76: 2364-2372.

Bouziane M, et al. (1994). Dietary protein deficiency affects n-3 and n-6 polyunsaturated fatty acids hepatic storage and very low density lipoprotein trasport in rats on different diets. Lipids 29(4): 265-272.

Brandi G, et al. (1996). Bacteria in biopsies of human hypochlorhydric stomach: a scanning electron microscopy study. Ultrastruct Pathol 20(3): 203-209.

Broadhurst CL (1997). Balanced intakes of natural triglycerides for optimum nutrition: an evolutionary and phytochemical perspective. Med Hypotheses 49(3): 247-261.

Buller R, et al. (1989). Specificity of lactate response in panic disorder, panic with concurrent depression and major depression. J Affective Dis 16: 109-113.

Butterfield GE (1987). Whole-body protein utilization in humans. Med Sci Sports Exerc 19(5): 157-165.

Cao G, et al. (1997). Antioxidant and pro-oxidant behavior of flavonoids: structure-activity relationships. Free Radic Biol Med 22(5): 749-760.

Castell L, et al. (1996). Does glutamine have a role in reducing infections in athletes? Eur J Appl Physiol 73(5): 488-90.

Champagne ET (1989). Low gastric hydrochloric acid secretion and mineral bioavailability. Adv Exp Med Biol 249: 173-184.

Chan MM, et al. (1995). Effects of three dietary phytochemicals from tea, rosemary and turmeric on inflammation-induced nitrite production. Cancer Lett 96(1): 23-29.

Christensen L, Somers S (1996). Comparison of nutrient intake among depressed and non-depressed individuals. Int J Eat Disord 20(1): 105-109.

Claassen N, et al. (1995). The effect of different n-6/n-3 essential fatty acid ratios on calcium balance and bone in rats. Prostaglandins Leukot Essent Fatty Acids 53: 13-19.

Clarkson PM (1995). Micronutrients and exercise: antioxidants and minerals. J Sports Sci 13 :S11-S24.

Convertino VA, et al. (1996). American College of Sports Medicine position stand. Exercise and fluid replacement. Med Sci Sports Exerc 28(1): I-VII.

Coulston AM, et al. (1993). Plasma glucose, insulin and lipid responses to high-carbohydrate low-fat diets in normal humans. Metabolism 32: 52-56.

Craig WJ (1997). Phytochemicals: guardians of our health. J Am Diet Assoc 10(2): S199-S204.

Cummings JH, Macfarlane GT (1997). Role of intestinal bacteria in nutrient metabolism. J Parenter Enteral Nutr 21(6):357-365.

Dekkers JC, et al. (1996). The role of antioxidant vitamins and enzymes in the prevention of exercise-induced muscle damage. Sports Med 21(3): 213-238.

Demopoulos H (1993). The development of secondary pathology with free radical reactions as a threshold mechanism. J Am Coll Toxicol 2: 173-184.

Desimone DP, et al. (1993). Prostaglandin E2 administered by subcutaneous pellets causes local inflammation and systemic bone loss: a model for inflammation-induced bone disease. J Bone Miner Res 8(5):625-634.

Deuster PA, et al. (1986). Nutritional intakes and status of highly trained amenorrheic and eumenorrheic women runners. Fertil Steril 46: 636-643.

Doucet E, Tremblay A (1997). Food intake, energy balance and body weight control. Eur J Clin Nutr 51(12): 846-855.

Dreon DM, et al. (1997). LDL subclass patterns and lipoprotein response to a low-fat, high-carbohydrate diet in women. Arterioscler Thromb Vasc Biol 17(4): 707-714.

REFERENCES

Drews L, et al. (1979). Effect of dietary fiber on copper, zinc, and magnesium utilization by adolescent boys. Am J Clin Nutr 32(9): 1893-1897.

Duchman S, et al. (1997). Upper limit for intestinal absorption of a dilute glucose solution in men at rest. Med Sci Sports Exerc 29(4): 482-488.

Dudkin M, et al. (1997). Dietary fibers as radiation protectors. Vopr Pitan 2: 12-14.

El-Sayed H, Hainsworth R (1996). Salt supplement increases plasma volume and orthostatic tolerance in patients with unexplained syncope. Heart 75(2): 134-140.

Enright T (1996). Exercise-induced asthma and the asthmatic athlete. Wis Med J 95(6): 375-378.

Expert panel on detection, evaluation, and treatment of high blood cholesterol in adults (1994). The second report of the National Cholesterol Education Program (NCEP) expert panel on detection, evaluation, and treatment of high blood cholesterol in adults. Circulation. 89: 1239-1445.

Fern EB, et al. (1991). Effects of exaggerated amino acid and protein supply in man. Experientia 47: 168-172.

Ferraris RP (1997). Effect of aging and caloric restriction on intestinal sugar and amino acid transport. Front Biosci 2: E108-E115.

Fiocchi A, et al. (1986). A double-blind clinical trial for the evaluation of the therapeutical effectiveness of a calf thymus derivative (Thymomodulin) in children with recurrent respiratory infections. Thymus 8(6): 331-339.

Foster C, et al. (1979). Effects of pre-exercise feedings on endurance performance. Med Sci Sports Exer 11(1); 1-5.

Foster-Powell K, Miller JB (1995). International tables of glycemic index. Am J Clin Nutr 62: 871S-893S.

Friedman JE, Lemon PWR (1989). Effect of chronic endurance exercise on retention of dietary protein. Int J Sports Med 10(2): 118-123.

Frizzell RT et al. (1986). Hyponatremia and ultramarathon running. JAMA 255: 772-774.

Gallaher DD, Schneeman BO. 1996. Dietary fiber. In Present knowledge in nutrition, ed. EE Ziegler and LJ Filer Jr. Washington DC: International Life Sciences Institute.

Gaur SN, et al. (1997). Use of LPC antagonist, choline, in the management of bronchial asthma. Indian J Chest Dis Allied Sci 39(2): 107-113.

Golay A, et al. (1996). Weight-loss with low or high carbohydrate diet? Int J Obes Relat Metab Disord 20(12): 1067-1072.

Goldfarb AH (1992). Antioxidants: role of supplementation to prevent exercise-induced oxidative stress. Med Sci Sports Exerc 25(2): 232-236.

Graham TE, Spriet LL (1995). Metabolic, catecholamine, and exercise performance responses to various doses of caffeine. J Appl Physiol 78(3): 867-874.

Granner DK. 1993. Hormones of the pancreas & gastrointestinal tract. In Harper's Biochemistry, eds. R.K. Murry, D.K. Granner, P.A. Mayes, V.W. Rodwell, pp. 563-564. Norwalk, CT: Appleton & Lange.

Graziani G, et al. (1995). Effect of gastric acid secretion on intestinal phosphate and calcium absorption in normal subjects. Nephrol Dial Transplant 10(8): 1376-1380.

Griffiths, AJ, et al. (1994). Forearm substrate utilization during exercise after a meal containing both fat and carbohydrate. Clinical Science 86: 169-175.

Gronbaek M, et al. (1995). Mortality associated with moderate intakes of wine, beer, or spirits. Br Med J 310: 1165-1169.

Grundy SM. 1996. Dietary Fat. In Present knowledge in nutrition, ed. EE Ziegler and LJ Filer Jr., p 44-57. Washington DC: International Life Sciences Institute.

Grynberg A, Demaison L (1996). Fatty acid oxidation in the heart. J. Cardiovasc Pharmacol 28(1): S11-S17.

Gupta SK; Gaur SN (1997). A placebo controlled trial of two dosages of LPC antagonist--choline in the management of bronchial asthma.

Indian J Chest Dis Allied Sci 39(3): 149-156.

Halliwell 1996. Antioxidants. In Present knowledge in nutrition, ed. EE Ziegler and LJ Filer Jr., p 596-603. Washington DC: International Life Sciences Institute.

Halstead CH. 1996. Alcohol: Medical and nutritional effects. In Present knowledge in nutrition, ed. EE Ziegler and LJ Filer Jr., p 547-556. Washington DC: International Life Sciences Institute.

Harper AE, Peters JC (1989). Protein intake, brain amino acid and serotonin concentrations and protein self-selection. J Nutr 119: 677-689.

Hawkins CL, Davies MJ (1997). Oxidative damage to collagen and related substrates by metal ion/hydrogen peroxide systems: random attack or site-specific damage? Biochem Biophys Acta 1360(1): 84-96.

Hawley JA, et al. (1997). Effects of 3 days of carbohydrate supplementation on muscle glycogen content and utilisation during a 1-h cycling performance. Eur J Appl Physiol 75(5):407-412.

Hirokawa K (1997). Reversing and restoring immune function. Mech Aging Dev 93(1-3): 119-124.

Hirokawa K, et al. (1992). Aging and immunity. Acta Pathol Jpn 42(8): 537-548.

Holder MD, DiBattista D (1994). Effects of time-restricted access to protein and of oral-sensory cues on protein selection. Physiol Behav 55(4): 659-664.

Holt S, et al. (1992). Relationship of satiety to postprandial glycaemic, insulin and cholecystokinin responses. Appetite 18: 129-141.

Houglum K, et al. (1997). Excess iron induces hepatic oxidative stress and transforming growth factor beta1 in genetic hemochromatosis. Hepatology 26(3): 605-610.

Islam S, et al. (1997). Glutamine is superior to glucose in stimulating water and electrolyte absorption across rabbit ileum. Dig Dis Sci 42(2): 420-423.

Ivaturi R, Kies C (1992). Mineral balances in humans as affected by fructose, high fructose corn syrup and sucrose. Plant Foods Hum Nutr 42(2): 143-151.

Jacobs I, et al. (1982). Dietary effects on glycogen and lipoprotein lipase activity in skeletal muscle in man. Acta Physiol Scand 115: 85-90.

Jacobson BH, et al. (1992). Effect of caffeine on maximal strength and power in elite male athletes. Br J Sports Med 26(4): 276-280.

Jain P, Khanna NK (1981). Evaluation of anti-inflammatory and analgesic properties of L-glutamine. Agents Actions 11(3): 243-249.

Jenkins D (1997). Carbohydrate tolerance and food frequency. Br J Nutr 77 (Suppl 1): S71-S81.

Jeppesen J, et al. (1997). Effects of low-fat, high-carbohydrate diets on risk factors for ischemic heart disease in postmenopausal women. Am J Clin Nutr 65(4): 1027-1033.

Joannic JL, et al. (1997). How the degree of unsaturation of dietary fatty acids influences the glucose and insulin responses to different carbohydrates in mixed meals. Am J Clin Nutr 65: 1427-1433.

Kamal-Eldin A, Appelqvist L (1996). The chemistry and antioxidant properties of tocopherols and tocotrienols. Lipids 31: 671-707.

Kamal-Eldin A, et al. (1995). Sesamin (a compound from sesame oil) increases tocopherol levels in rats fed ad libitum. Lipids 30(6): 499-505.

Kelso TB, et al. (1989). Enzymes of glutamine metabolism in inflammation associated with skeletal muscle hypertrophy. Am J Physiol 257(6 Pt 1): E885-E894.

Kiens B, et al. (1987). Lipoprotein lipase activity and intramuscular triglyceride stores after long-term high-fat and high-carbohydrate diets in physically trained men. Clinical Physiol 7: 1-9.

Koester MC (1993). An overview of the physiology and pharmacology of aspirin and nonsteroidal anti-inflammatory drugs. J Athletic Training 28(3): 252-259.

Kreider RB, et al. (1993). Amino acid supplementation and exercise performance - analysis of the proposed ergogenic value. Sports Med 16: 190-209.

Lacey JM, Wilmore DW (1990). Is glutamine a conditionally essential amino acid? Nutrition Reviews 48(8): 233-245.

Lambert EV, et al. (1994). Enhanced endurance in trained cyclists during moderate intensity exercise following 2 weeks adaptation to a high fat diet. Eur J Appl Physiol 69: 287-293.

Larue-Achagiotis C, et al. (1992). Dietary self-selection vs. complete diet: body weight gain and meal pattern in rats. Physiol Behav 51(5): 995-999.

Lehmann M, et al. (1993). Serum amino acid concentrations in nine athletes before and after the 1993 Colmar ultra triathlon. Int J Sports Med 16(3):155-159.

Lemon PW (1996). Is increased dietary protein necessary or beneficial for individuals with a physically active lifestyle? Nutr Rev 54(4 Pt 2): S169-175.

Liu GC, et al. (1983). Effect of high-carbohydrate-low-fat diets on plasma glucose, insulin and lipid responses in hypertriglyceridemic humans. Metabolism 32(8): 750-753.

Luft FC. 1996. Salt, water and extracellular volume regulation. In Present knowledge in nutrition, ed. EE Ziegler and LJ Filer Jr., p 265. Washington DC: International Life Sciences Institute.

Lukaski HC, et al. (1996). Iron, copper magnesium and zinc status as predictors of swimming performance. Int J Sports Med 17(7): 535-540.

MacLaren D, et al. (1994). Hormonal and metabolic responses to glucose and maltodextrin ingestion with or without the addition of guar gum. Int. J. Sports Med 15: 466-471.

Martinsen E, et al. (1989). Physical fitness level in patients with anxiety and depressive disorders. Int. J. Sports Med 10(1): 58-61.

Massey L, et al. (1994). Interactions between dietary caffeine and calcium on calcium and bone metabolism in older women. J Am Coll Nutr 13(6): 592-596.

Massicotte D, et al. (1989). Oxidation of a glucose polymer during exercise: comparison with glucose and fructose. J Appl Physiol 66(1): 179-183.

Mattes RD (1997). Physiologic responses to sensory stimulation by food: nutritional implications. J Am Diet Assoc 97(4):406-413.

Maughan RJ., et al. (1997). Factors influencing the restoration of fluid and electrolyte balance after exercise in the heat. Br J Sports Med 31(3): 175-182.

McNamara DJ, et al. (1987). Heterogeneity of cholesterol homeostatis in man. Response to changes in dietary fat quality and cholesterol quantity. J Clin Invest 79(6): 1729-1739.

Meredith CN, et al. (1992). Body composition in elderly men: effect of dietary modification during strength training. J Am Ger Soc 40: 155-162.

Mero A; et al. (1997). Leucine supplementation and serum amino acids, testosterone, cortisol and growth hormone in male power athletes during training. J Sports Med Phys Fitness 37(2): 137-45.

Messina M, Messina V (1996). Nutritional implications of dietary phytochemicals. Adv Exp Med Biol; 401:207-212.

Miller CC, Tang W, Ziboh VA, Fletcher MP (1991). Dietary supplementation with ethyl ester concentrates of fish oil (n-3) and borage oil (n-6) polyunsaturated fatty acids induces epidermal generation of local putative anti-inflammatory metabolites. J Invest Dermatol 96(1): 98-103.

Miller WC, et al. (1984). Adaptations to a high-fat diet that increase exercise endurance in male rats. J Appl Physiol 56(1): 78-83.

Miyajima H, et al. (1989). Muscle carnitine deficiency associated with myalgia and rhabdomyolysis following exercise. Rinsho Shinkeigaku 29(1): 93-97.

Moller P, et al. (1996). Oxidative stress associated with exercise, psychological stress and life-style factors. Chem Biol Interact 102(1): 17-36.

Moore CE, et al. (1983). The relationship of exercise and diet on HDL cholesterol levels in women. Metabolism 32(2): 189-196.

Muoio DM, et al. (1994). Effect of dietary fat on metabolic adjustments to maximal VO2 and endurance in runners. Med Sci Sports Exerc 26(1): 81-88.

Murray R, et al. (1994). Gastric emptying of water and isocaloric carbohydrate solutions consumed at rest. Med Sci. Sports Exerc 26(6): 725-732.

Nestel PJ (1993). Contribution of fats and fatty acids to performance of the elite athlete. In Simopoulos AP, Pavlou KN (eds.): Nutrition and fitness for athletes. World Rev Nutr Diet Basel, Karger 71: 61-68.

Newsholme EA (1994). Biochemical mechanisms to explain immunosuppression in well-trained and overtrained athletes. Int J Sports Med 15: S142-S147.

Noakes TD (1992). The hyponatremia of exercise. Int J Sport Nutr 2(3): 205-228.

Nutter J (1991). Seasonal changes in female athlete's diets. Int J Sport Nutr. 1(4): 395-407.

Packer L (1997). Oxidants, antioxidant nutrients and the athlete. J Sports Sci 15(3): 353-363.

Pan DA, Lillioja S, et al. (1995). Skeletal muscle membrane lipid composition is related to adiposity and insulin action. J Clin Invest 96: 2802-2808.

Parker LN, Levin ER, Lifrak ET (1985). Evidence for adrenocortical adaptation to severe illness. J Clin Endocrinol Metab 60: 947-952.

Parry-Billings M, et al. (1992). Plasma amino acid concentrations in the overtraining syndrome: possible effects on the immune system. Med Sci Sports Exerc 24(12): 1353-1358.

Pendergast DR, et al. (1996). The role of dietary fat on performance, metabolism and health. Am J Sports Med 24(6): S53-S58.

Pyne DB (1994). Exercise-induced muscle damage and inflammation: a review. Aust J Sci Med Sport 26(3-4): 49-58.

Rankin JW, et al. (1996). Effect of weight loss and refeeding diet composition on anaerobic performance in wrestlers. Med Sci Sports Exerc 28(10): 1292-1299.

Ravich WJ, et al. (1983). Fructose: incomplete intestinal absorption in humans. Gastroenterology 84(1):26-29.

Reaven GM (1997). Do high carbohydrate diets prevent the development or attenuate the manifestations (or both) of syndrome X? A viewpoint strongly against. Curr Opin Lipidol 8(1): 23-27.

Reed MJ, Cheng RW, Simmonds M, Richmond W, James VH (1987). Dietary lipids: an additional regulator of plasma levels of sex hormone binding globulin. J Clin Endocrinol Metab 64(5): 1083-1085.

Rieth N, Larue-Achagiotis C (1997). Exercise training decreases body fat more in self-selecting than in chow-fed rats. Physiol Behav 62(6): 1291-1297.

Rowbottom DG, Keast D, Morton AR (1996). The emerging role of glutamine as an indicator of exercise stress and overtraining. Sports Med 21(2): 80-97.

Salonen JT, et al. (1992). High stored iron levels are associated with excess risk of myocardial infarction in eastern Finnish men. Circulation 86: 803-811.

Savendahl L, et al. (1997). Prolonged fasting in humans results in diminished plasma choline concentrations but does not cause liver dysfunction. Am J Clin Nutr 66(3): 622-625.

Sawka MN, Greenleaf JE (1992). Current concepts concerning thirst, dehydration, and fluid replacement: overview. Med Sci Sports Exerc 24(6): 643-644.

Sigleo S, et al. (1984). Effects of dietary fiber constituents on intestinal morphology and nutrient transport. Am J Physiol 246 (1 Pt 1):G34-39.

Siguel EN, Lerman RH (1996). Prevelance of essential fatty acid deficiency in patients with chronic gastrointestinal disorders. Metabolism 45(1): 12-23.

Simi B, Sempore B, Mayet M, Favier RJ (1991). Additive effects of training and high-fat diet on energy metabolism during exercise. J Appl Physiol 71(1): 197-203.

Simopoulos AP (1991). Omega-3 fatty acids in health and disease and in growth and development. Am J Clin Nutr 54(3):438-463.

Skouby SO, et al. (1990). Mechanism of action of oral contraceptives on carbohydrate metabolism at the cellular level. Am J Obstet Gynecol 163: 343-348.

Snodgrass SR (1992). Vitamin neurotoxicity. Mol. Neurobiol. 6(1): 41-73.

Song MK, et al. (1998). Effects of bovine prostate powder on zinc, glucose, and insulin metabolism in old patients with non-insulin-dependent diabetes mellitus. Metabolism 47(1): 39-43.

Speedy DB, Faris JG, Hamlin M, Gallagher PG, Campbell RG (1997). Hyponatremia and weight changes in an ultradistance triathlon. Clin J Sport Med 7(3): 180-184.

Surgenor S, Uphold RE (1994). Acute hyponatremia in ultra-endurance athletes. Am. J Emerg Med 12(4): 441-444.

Takahashi O (1995). Haemorrhagic toxicity of a large dose of alpha-, beta-, gamma- and delta-tocopherols, ubiquinone, beta-carotene, retinol acetate and L-ascorbic acid in the rat. Food Chem Toxicol 33(2): 121-128.

Tarnopolsky MA, et al. (1992). Evaluation of protein requirements for trained strength athletes. J Appl Physiol 73: 1986-1995.

Tarnopolsky MA, et al. (1995). Carbohydrate loading and metabolism during exercise in men and women. J Appl Physiol 78(4):1360-1368.

Tarnopolsky MA, et al. (1997). Postexercise protein-carbohydrate and carbohydrate supplements increase muscle glycogen in men and women. J Appl Physiol 83(6): 1877-1883.

Thomas DE, et al. (1991). Carbohydrate feeding before exercise: effect of glycemic index. Int J Sports Med 12: 10-186.

Thomas DE, et al. (1994). Plasma glucose levels after prolonged strenuous exercise correlate inversely with glycemic response to food consumed before exercise. Int J Sports Nutr 4: 361-373.

Tilles S, et al. (1995). Exercise-induced anaphylaxis related to specific foods. J Pediatr 127(4): 587-589.

Torre M, et al. (1991). Effects of dietary fiber and phytic acid on mineral availability. Crit Rev Food Sci Nutr 1(1): 1-22.

Toth MJ, Poehlman ET (1994). Sympathetic nervous system activity and resting metabolic rate in vegetarians. Metabolism 43(5): 621-625.

Umeda-Sawada R, et al. (1995). Interaction of sesamin and eicosapentaenoic acid against delta 5 desaturation and n-6/n-3 ratio of essential fatty acids in rat. Biosci Biotechnol Biochem 59(12): 2268-2273.

van der Beek EJ (1991). Vitamin supplementation and physical exercise performance. J Sports Sci 9: 77-90.

van der Beek EJ, et al. (1988). Thiamin, riboflavin, and vitamins B-6 and C: impact of combined restricted intake on functional performance in man. Am J Clin Nutr 48: 1451-1462.

van der Beek EJ, et al. (1994). Thiamin, riboflavin and vitamin B6: impact of restricted intake on physical performance in man. J Am Coll Nutr 13(6): 629-640.

van der Hulst RR, et al. (1993). Glutamine and the preservation of gut integrity. Lancet 341(8857): 1363-1365.

Veera RK, et al. (1992). Exercise-induced oxidant stress in the lung tissue: role of dietary supplementation of vitamin E and selenium. Biochem Int 26(5): 863-871.

Venkatraman JT, et al. (1997). Influence of the level of dietary lipid intake and maximal exercise on the immune status in runners. Med Sci Sports Exerc 29(3): 333-344.

Vukovich MD, et al. (1993). Effect of fat emulsion infusion and fat feeding on muscle glycogen utilization during cycle exercise. J Appl Physiol 75(4): 1513-1518.

Wiles JD, Bet al. (1992). Effect of caffeinated coffee on running speed, respiratory factors, blood lactate and perceived exertion during 1500-m treadmill running. Br J Sports Med 26(2): 116-120.

Willi SM, et al. (1998). The Effects of a high-protein, low-fat, ketogenic diet on adolescents with morbid obesity. Pediatrics 101(1): 61-67.

Index

Other Books by the Author

"Training for Endurance"

David Barmore Productions

"In Fitness and In Health"

David Barmore Productions

"Complementary Sports Medicine"

textbook, Human Kinetics

"ABCs of Burning Body Fat"

booklet, David Barmore Productions

For information about ordering these books and many of the products mentioned in this book, including Phil's Bar, contact us at:

Toll-free: (877) 264-2200

E-mail: info@philsbar.com

Web site: www.philsbar.com